M000284849

**2017 2018**

SAUNDERS

Guide to Success in

# NURSING SCHOOL

## A Student PLANNER

**Holly Stromberg**, RN, BSN, MSN, PHN, CCRN

**Susan C. deWit**, MSN, RN, CNS, PHN

ELSEVIER

# ELSEVIER

3251 Riverport Lane
St. Louis, Missouri 63043

SAUNDERS GUIDE TO SUCCESS IN NURSING SCHOOL,
2017-2018: A STUDENT PLANNER, 13TH EDITION                    ISBN: 978-0-323-49750-3

**Copyright © 2018 by Elsevier, Inc. All rights reserved.**
**Copyright © 2017, 2016, 2015, 2014, 2013, 2012, 2010, 2007, 2006, 2003, 1999, 1995 by Saunders,**
**an imprint of Elsevier, Inc.**

No part of this publication may be reproduced or transmitted in any form or by any means, electronic or
mechanical, including photocopying, recording, or any information storage and retrieval system, without
permission in writing from the publisher. Details on how to seek permission, further information about the
Publisher's permissions policies and our arrangements with organizations such as the Copyright Clearance
Center and the Copyright Licensing Agency, can be found at our website: www.elsevier.com/permissions.

This book and the individual contributions contained in it are protected under copyright by the Publisher
(other than as may be noted herein).

---

### Notices

Knowledge and best practice in this field are constantly changing. As new research and experience
broaden our understanding, changes in research methods, professional practices, or medical treatment
may become necessary.

Practitioners and researchers must always rely on their own experience and knowledge in evaluating and using any information, methods, compounds, or experiments described herein. In using such
information or methods they should be mindful of their own safety and the safety of others, including
parties for whom they have a professional responsibility.

With respect to any drug or pharmaceutical products identified, readers are advised to check the
most current information provided (i) on procedures featured or (ii) by the manufacturer of each
product to be administered, to verify the recommended dose or formula, the method and duration
of administration, and contraindications. It is the responsibility of practitioners, relying on their own
experience and knowledge of their patients, to make diagnoses, to determine dosages and the best
treatment for each individual patient, and to take all appropriate safety precautions.

To the fullest extent of the law, neither the Publisher nor the authors, contributors, or editors,
assume any liability for any injury and/or damage to persons or property as a matter of products liability, negligence or otherwise, or from any use or operation of any methods, products, instructions, or
ideas contained in the material herein.

---

**Library of Congress Cataloging-in-Publication Data**

Names: deWit, Susan C., author. | Stromberg, Holly, author.
Title: Saunders guide to success in nursing school : 2017-2018 : a student
    planner / Holly Stromberg, Susan C. deWit.
Other titles: Saunders guide to success in nursing school 2016-2017 | Guide
    to success in nursing school : 2017-2018
Description: 13th edition. | St. Louis, Missouri : Elsevier, 2017. | Preceded
    by Saunders guide to success in nursing school 2016-2017 / Susan C. deWit.
    12th edition. [2017] | Susan C. deWit's name appears first in the previous
    edition. | Includes bibliographical references and index.
Identifiers: LCCN 2017001874 | ISBN 9780323497503 (paperback) | ISBN
    9780323533713 (e-ISBN)
Subjects: | MESH: Nursing Process | Patient Care Planning | Medical Records |
    Students, Nursing
Classification: LCC RT73 | NLM WY 100 | DDC 610.73076--dc23 LC record
    available at https://lccn.loc.gov/2017001874

*Senior Content Strategist:* Nancy O'Brien
*Content Development Manager:* Ellen Wurm-Cutter
*Associate Content Development Specialist:* Erin Garner
*Publishing Services Manager:* Deepthi Unni
*Senior Project Manager:* Kamatchi Madhavan
*Design Direction:* Patrick Ferguson

Printed in the United States of America

Last digit is the print number: 9  8  7  6  5  4  3  2  1

Working together
to grow libraries in
developing countries

www.elsevier.com • www.bookaid.org

To

**Susan C. deWit**

educator, author, nurse, mentor, and friend.
This planner and many other publications exist due to
Susan's dedication to producing a quality product that
is current, accurate and student friendly.
She has made a great contribution to nursing education
by her tireless efforts. Susan, thank you for sharing your
wisdom and for your friendship. You are appreciated.

# PREFACE

The student nursing experience is one of the most complex in the undergraduate curriculum. It entails not only the class work and home study common to all undergraduate programs but also unique clinical preparations and experiences. In talking with students, nursing program administrators, and nursing classroom and clinical instructors, we found that people were looking for a guide to help students plan and organize their time and information, particularly with respect to the clinical experience. Much of the material in this book is for quick reference throughout the nursing program and during clinical experiences.

## ■ CLINICAL INFORMATION

Chapters 1 through 6 of this planner include an orientation to and a guide for success throughout your nursing program, including suggestions for getting the most from clinical rotations, achieving success in distance learning courses, and dealing with stress and a broad array of useful data and procedures. The information in this section was selected especially for student use in a quick reference format and has been indexed for user convenience.

## ■ CALENDARS

Yearly, monthly, and weekly calendars have been included so that students can plan their short-term weekly activities and long-term projects and goals.

# CONTENTS

# 5 CLINICAL QUICK REFERENCE 82

# SUCCESS IN NURSING SCHOOL

## ■ QUALIFICATIONS AND PREPARATION

Nursing schools generally have prerequisite courses that must be passed before entry into the nursing program. Other entrance requirements may also be necessary. Check with your school regarding the requirements and scheduling of the required courses.

Specific regulations and requirements exist for any person who has had a criminal conviction or been treated for a psychiatric occurrence. **It is wise to check with your state board of nursing before beginning the nursing program or during the first course to review these regulations and requirements.** Even juvenile offenses are not sealed to the board of nursing. Licensure may be denied because of past offenses that are "substantially related to health care" or exhibit a lack of integrity, such as bouncing checks or shoplifting. If there is a past history of criminal offenses, character references may counter juvenile offenses.

Clinical agencies require a background check that includes drug screening, as for all employees and volunteers, before a student is allowed into the clinical area. Failing the background check may exclude you from clinical courses and delay your entry into the nursing program.

## ■ ETHICS AND PROFESSIONALISM

In its *Code of Ethics for Nurses with Interpretive Statements*, the American Nurses Association (ANA) states, "Inherent in professional nursing is a process of education and formation. That process involves the ongoing acquisition and development of the knowledge, skills, dispositions, practice experiences, commitment, relational maturity, and personal integrity essential for professional practice" (ANA, 2015). Nursing students are expected to act ethically **at all times**. Acting ethically includes being honest with your written work and tests and following the policies of the institution in which you are a student. It means protecting the privacy and well-being of your patient at all times with adherence to the Health Insurance Portability and Accountability Act (HIPAA) privacy law. Acting ethically also relates to your **personal** life as well. It is important to act with integrity and pay attention to what you say and do.

*Professionalism* means that you act decorously, with good manners, and treat others courteously. An example is to change out of your uniform before going out with friends after clinical or work for drinks or boisterous activity. When blogging or commenting on social networking sites, remember that what you post is no longer in your control and can be seen by anyone. Privacy settings on social networking sites are easy to circumvent and are often changed by web administrators without notice. It is possible that the information you thought you were sharing only with close friends has been viewed by teachers and prospective employers.

It is not appropriate to use these venues for venting about school issues or other people. It is not professional to use coarse language orally or in writing on social networking sites. **Employers often check these sites to gather data about the character of prospective employees.** A guide to basic good manners is available at http://www.nursingcenter.com/lnc/journalarticle?Article_ID=983314.

## ■ CHALLENGES OF NURSING SCHOOL

Nursing school is an exciting and challenging adventure that demands significant time and energy. Because nursing is a discipline comprising knowledge from many related fields, you are asked to learn to think critically, synthesize information, and then apply this information to everyday situations involving people. To learn to care correctly and safely for people who are ill, you must learn a large amount of information in a relatively short time. This process requires an efficient use of time and resources.

### On Campus

#### SYLLABUS

A course outline or syllabus will be provided for each nursing course (Fig. 1.1). This outline or syllabus may be available on the college learning management system (LMS) for you to download and print or available for purchase in the bookstore or handed out in class. Becoming familiar with the entire layout of each course is the first step after you acquire the syllabus. Syllabi, or course outlines, are usually divided into units of study that contain a list of learning objectives. A correlated outline of the content to be covered in the unit and related learning opportunities or activities may also be provided. The latter usually includes textbook and journal reading assignments, electronic media or online instruction modules, clinical simulations, and suggestions for review of material covered in earlier prerequisite classes, such as anatomy and physiology.

The syllabus, or other class materials (student handbook) available electronically or handed out at the first class meeting, will state policies regarding attendance requirements, student behavior in class and clinical areas, grading criteria, dress code for clinical areas, grievance procedures, and other topics. A list of required texts and a statement about evaluation of performance for the course will be provided. Many schools are switching to electronic textbooks and therefore require students to have an iPad, tablet, or other electronic device to access texts. Most print texts have online electronic resources requiring Internet access and a device for connecting.

#### SCHOOL PHILOSOPHY AND STUDENT RESPONSIBILITY

Each school and nursing program has a statement of philosophy that explains how the school and instructors view the student, the teacher, and learning. Most schools expect the student to be an active learner and the teacher to be a facilitator of learning. This means that you must take responsibility for your own learning and must not depend on instructors to provide all the knowledge you need to pass a particular course. You are expected to participate in all classroom and lab activities.

For this reason, going to class prepared for the topics to be covered that day is very important. You are properly prepared if all assigned learning activities have been completed: you have read the text pages relative to the content to be covered, taken study notes, considered the objectives to be covered, viewed voice-over

Sample Page from a Nursing Course Syllabus

| Content Outline | Learning Objectives | Assignment | Learning Resources |
|---|---|---|---|
| Unit 2 Assessment<br>A. Introduction<br>B. History taking<br>  1. History of current<br>    problems<br>  2. Medical history<br>  3. Psychosocial data<br>C. Physical assessment<br>  1. Assessment techniques<br>    a. Observation<br>    b. Palpation<br>    c. Percussion<br>    d. Auscultation<br>    e. Olfaction<br>  2. Height and weight<br>  3. Neurologic<br>    assessment<br>    a. Level of<br>      consciousness<br>    b. Pupillary response<br>    c. Motor/sensory<br>      response<br>  4. Vital sign trends<br>  5. Testing visual acuity<br>  5. Assisting for a medical<br>    exam<br>    a. Positioning<br>    b. Draping | 1. Demonstrate methods for obtaining a health history from a patient.<br><br>2. Describe the steps in performing a chart review.<br><br>3. Identify techniques used for obtaining physical assessment data.<br><br>4. List the equipment needed for a complete physical assessment.<br><br>5. Correctly demonstrate a basic neurologic assessment.<br><br>6. Identify indications of a patient problem from vital sign trends.<br><br>7. Prepare a patient for a medical physical examination, including a rectal and pelvic examination. | deWit Fundamentals Chapters 21 and 22<br><br>Potter & Perry Skills & Techniques Chapters 17 and 18<br><br>Simulation practice in Skill Lab | Evolve text website<br>Video clips<br>Mosby's Nursing Skills<br>  Video Exercises<br><br>Mosby's Nursing Skills<br>Video/CD-ROM:<br>Measurements Video: Height and weight; intake and output; vital signs.<br><br>Norton, C., Feltz, S., Brocker, A., Granitto, M. (2016) Tackling long-term consequences of concussion, *Nursing2016* 43(1), p. 50-55 |

**FIG. 1.1** Sample page from a nursing course syllabus.

Microsoft PowerPoint or recorded lectures on the LMS if available, and noted questions that should be asked in class.

Students who use English as a second language must be able to read and write in English by writing or printing on paper as well as by computer keyboard.

During orientation to each course, the calendar of when course material will be covered by date will be given. Test dates and assignment due dates will also be set. Enter this information in the Monthly Calendar section of this planner or into a tablet or smartphone calendar. Doing so assists in organizing time and study activity.

## CAMPUS RESOURCES

Become acquainted with the resources on campus that can make life easier. All nursing students have access to the learning resource center or library. Your campus might also have a learning or tutoring center, adult resource center for single parents or students with special needs, office for students with disabilities, counseling center, computer lab, testing center, media room, skills and simulation lab, and student center. The school catalog or student handbook describes these areas and services. Plan time to seek out, visit, and use the services and areas that could be useful to you. You are entitled to the services offered through the tuition and fees paid for courses. Your school may have a bulletin board that features important announcements and reminders for nursing students.

You should become familiar with the school LMS, where syllabi, class notes, instructions, announcements for class, and other information may be posted. The LMS software (Blackboard, WebCT, Canvas, E-College, etc.) that the school uses should have a tutorial available to help you navigate the site and areas within it that you will need.

Schedule time each week for working with campus resources, using available media, participating in computer or mannequin simulations, and practicing skills. Few schools can schedule sufficient lab time for students to learn a skill thoroughly or provide adequate practice time to master a skill. **You are expected to practice on your own time.** Schedule these activities each week in the Monthly Calendar section of this planner. Practice with a peer and, when the skill is mastered, ask your peer to evaluate your performance critically. Peer evaluation will help ensure that you are ready for instructor "check-off" evaluation.

## SKILL LAB OR SIMULATION PRACTICE

You should prepare for lab time by studying the assigned skill before coming to the lab. If media presentations are available, use them. Be attentive to instruction in the lab, and practice the skill using a guide and a partner to check your technique. There may be a pretest and then a post-test for the exercises or scenarios.

A simulation experience with a mannequin may take the place of some clinical hours and is just as serious a learning experience as clinical experience with a real patient. The mannequins are programmed to react to a given situation or problem much like a person would react. You are expected to treat the simulation mannequin as you would a real human. To prepare for a simulation assignment, you should find out the following:

- Are there preparation assignments?
- What are the objectives for the experience?
- What is the dress code?

- What kind of orientation to the equipment will be given?
- What should you bring to the simulation area?
- Will the simulation exercise be recorded?
- Is confidentiality about the simulation exercise required?

### At the Hospital

The term *clinical* refers to the time you are scheduled to learn at the hospital or another clinical site. When you have learned the preliminary skills necessary to function in the clinical area, you will be assigned to a clinical facility. Hospitals, long-term care facilities (nursing homes), mental health facilities, home health agencies, rehabilitation facilities, school health offices, and outpatient clinics are all referred to as *clinical facilities*. Clinical rotations may be for 1, 2, or 3 days, a few weeks, half of a semester, or a full semester. Sometimes night or weekend shift times are assigned. Once assigned to a clinical facility, you may be given data about the type of patient assignment the day before the clinical experience is to take place. Otherwise, specific patients are assigned at the beginning of the clinical session.

Hospital rules usually require that tattoos and piercing jewelry not be visible on student nurses. Cell phone use on the units is governed by facility policy and may be restricted to contacting your instructor for assistance. Only the items you need for your clinical assignment are to be brought into the hospital. Because lockers are not usually available for students, purses, backpacks, and other personal items should be locked in the trunk of your vehicle. The hospital usually insists on photo ID and may take your picture for your badge that will give you access to the units to which your clinical group is assigned.

### CLINICAL ORIENTATION

During clinical orientation you will be given an overview of the facility, including its size, general services, and the community it serves; whether the facility is a public or private business; its administrative structure; the physical layout; and the areas to which you will be assigned. A description of the type of nursing care used on the units will be provided. Some hospitals use a team nursing approach, some use managed care, and others use primary nursing; many different types of care delivery exist. (The types of care delivery are discussed further in your fundamentals of nursing course.) Importantly, you must understand the division of labor among the personnel on the unit, the organization of the unit, and the lines of communication. **Note that the patient, or client, is considered the customer and is to be treated as such.**

A clinical facility orientation checklist is provided to help you prepare to care for patients and to feel more comfortable in the environment of the assigned clinical unit (Box 1.1). This checklist is most appropriate for a hospital unit, but it can be adapted to other types of clinical facilities. Authorization for electronic health record (EHR) access is usually obtained during the orientation period; it may take several days to process requests. EHR training may be included as part of orientation. Implementation of EHRs is a federal mandate, which means that facilities will use electronic rather than paper medical records. Most facilities have made this transition. Students must become adept at accessing information about their patients via computer.

### PATIENT ASSIGNMENT

During clinical orientation, your instructor will describe how you will receive your patient assignments for the clinical days; either your instructor will assign patients

## Clinical Facility Orientation

BOX 1.1

### TOUR THE FACILITY
- Find out where you should park and which door you should enter.
- Identify where the cafeteria or eating area is located.
- Locate central supply, lab, pharmacy, and imaging departments.
- Determine the location and type of unit of your assignment.

### MEET THE PERSONNEL AND FACILITY DEPARTMENTS
Find out how to access the internal phone directory for phone numbers of essential people and departments. Have immediately available the following:

- Unit director's or charge nurse's name (or both) and contact information
- Instructor (cell or pager)
- Pharmacy
- Imaging department (x-ray, MRI, ultrasound)
- Respiratory therapy department
- Central supply or central stores

### EQUIPMENT
- Learn to work the intercom system if students are allowed to use it.
- Use colored light system or other types of designations for special patient needs.
- Review the procedure for using the fire extinguishers and note alarm locations.
- Proceed to a patient unit and perform the following:
  - Operate all of the light switches.
  - Turn the television on and off, and adjust the volume; use the other functions of the control unit. Note patient education programs available within the facility and how to show them to patients.
  - Identify the resources for language interpretation (usually via the telephone).
  - Raise and lower the whole bed; raise the head and then the foot.
  - Raise and lower the side rails.
  - Open and close the curtains or blinds.
  - Practice using the call-light system.
  - Adjust the shower or bath controls.

### ENVIRONMENT
- Explore the layout of the nurses' station, and find extra forms if the system is not paperless.
- Find items you may need during a clinical day:
  - Chart rack (even if EHR is used, there is usually a place for any paper to be kept prior to scanning into the electronic record)
  - Kardex or computer patient care sheets
  - Drug reference access
  - Policy and procedure manuals
  - Dietary manual
  - Communication board
  - Out-of-the-way areas where students can sit to chart
  - Location of computers for documentation and access to the Internet and clinical agency system
  - Location of shred containers for disposal of items with patient information
- Find all supplies that you may need for patient care; explore the supply cart and various cupboards.
- Find the clean linen storage area.
- Locate the dirty linen disposal area and the utility room.

## Clinical Facility Orientation (cont'd)

- Locate the lift equipment locations.
- Find the staff restroom.
- Locate the patient shower or tub bathrooms if such exist on the unit.
- Find the room or area where reports are given.
- Determine where to leave your coat.
- Find out how student–patient assignments are identified.

### PROCEDURES

- Learn how to access patient data in the EHR, if permitted.
- Determine how to document care (check the documentation policies).
- Understand the fire and disaster procedures.
- Learn the procedure for initiating the code for cardiac or respiratory emergencies.
- Learn how to activate the rapid response team.
- Determine how to handle hazardous materials.
- Understand the procedures for obtaining supplies for patient care and any method for charging for supplies and equipment used.
- Learn the policies for administering medication and to use the medication-dispensing machine or medication retrieval system.
- Understand the procedure for charting as-needed (*pro re nata* [PRN]) medications and one-time doses.
- Learn the narcotic checkout procedure and/or the use of the automated dispensing machine.
- Understand the special charting and reporting procedures (e.g., abnormal vital signs, change in condition).

to you or you will choose your own patients. In either case, you will need to gather data to prepare for your patient assignment. Box 1.2 provides a checklist for you to use to be certain you gather the essential information.

### HEAVILY TRAFFICKED AREAS

During orientation you should pay attention to heavily trafficked areas to avoid obstructing the work of the unit. Heavily traveled pathways and chairs where nurses or physicians need to sit to document should be avoided at peak times of the day. Consideration will be appreciated. If the facility has not completely changed to EHRs and is using paper charts, whenever a chart is taken away from the immediate area of the nurses' station, inform the unit secretary where the chart will be in case someone needs it. Charts must be replaced exactly where they were found.

Take note of particular landmarks on the way to the assigned unit if the facility is large or the layout is confusing. Try to travel to and from the unit on the same elevators each time, and note hallway decor and signs with unit and room number designations.

Some instructors will assign you to a staff nurse the first day of clinical orientation to ensure that you can become more comfortable and learn the usual routine of the unit.

### PRECONFERENCE AND POSTCONFERENCE

Many schools have a preconference period at the beginning of the clinical day to provide an opportunity for students to clarify assignments, ask questions, and

## Clinical Assignment Information Form

BOX 1.2

- Age and length of stay
- Diagnoses
- Surgery and date performed
- Current vital signs and condition; vital sign schedule
- Current pertinent lab values
- Daily weight required
- Type of diet:
  - Intake and output (I&O)
  - Any swallowing difficulty
- Activity allowed:
  - Degree of mobility
  - Traction
- Type of bath needed
- Tubes:
  - Intravenous (IV) peripheral or central line
  - Nasogastric (NG) tube
  - Foley catheter
  - Drains
  - Other
- Pain:
  - Control method
  - Pain score
- Medications
- Allergies
- Risk areas:
  - Skin
  - Falls
- Treatments:
  - Dressing changes
  - Thromboembolic deterrent: anticoagulants, sequential compression devices (SCDs)
  - Incentive spirometer
  - Turn, cough, and deep breathe (TCDB)
- Therapies:
  - Physical
  - Occupational
  - Respiratory
  - Speech
- Tests ordered
- Equipment in use
- Prostheses
- Losses:
  - Hearing
  - Vision (wears glasses or contact lenses)
  - Paralysis or limb weakness
- Communication:
  - Problems
  - Language spoken
- Treatment plan – goals for the day

gather moral support for the day. At the end of the clinical day, most schools have a 30-minute to several-hour clinical postconference time for discussion of the day's events, sharing of experiences, and instructor-guided learning to help meet the week's objectives. Students are often asked to make presentations on short topics, complete quizzes, or participate in group learning activities. Sometimes speakers are invited to present special topics to the clinical group.

## NETWORKING

You should begin networking with classmates and other nursing students as soon as school starts. Networking will help you find out what to expect in other courses, at particular clinical facilities, and from particular instructors. Networking is also a way to develop study buddies and to set up a study group. Online groups of student nurses provide a social network for those with little time to socialize otherwise. Be very careful in using social media as a mechanism for networking. Joining the student nurses' association (SNA) at your school is one way to begin. Your instructors can provide you with information about SNA meetings and contact information for sponsors and officers.

# ■ SETTING UP FOR SUCCESS

Being successful in nursing school requires good time management, efficient study skills, and proper use of appropriate resources. Nursing students often have to juggle family responsibilities, work, and school, along with the miscellaneous tasks of daily life. **The key to success is careful planning and as much simplification as possible in all areas of your life for the duration of the nursing program.** Besides the hours spent in class and in clinical settings, a rule of thumb for planning study time is 2 hours per week for each credit hour of the course to achieve a passing grade. In other words, for a 3-credit-hour course, you will need to spend 6 hours studying per week to obtain a C average.

## Organizing Your Time

### WEEKLY TIME MAP

Coordinating all of your responsibilities and activities of day-to-day life with your school class and study schedule is essential to your success in any nursing program. Making a weekly time map in which you map out the time required for everything from cooking dinner or mowing the yard to picking up the children from school is a good way to coordinate all responsibilities and activities. The student living alone will want to coordinate time for friends, exercise, and favorite pastimes with the school schedule. The student living with family will want to set aside some time to spend with family members. Fig. 1.2 illustrates one student's time map for 1 week. Fig. 1.3 provides an example of a blank time map.

Use a pencil when creating your time map, because your first estimates may not work. Adjust the schedule until it is more accurate for each activity, and do not forget to include at least a little time for the important people in your life and leisure time for yourself. Nothing but work and study may lead to burnout before the nursing program is completed. Enter all firm commitments, study times, time for completing assignments, and appointments in the calendar in this planner. Schedule class and study time on the time map first, working personal and social activities around them. Scheduling keeps your social time from interfering with sufficient study and sets you up for success in your nursing program. Using an electronic calendar in Microsoft Outlook, Gmail, Yahoo!, or your smartphone or other device is also advised. You will be sent reminders that you've programmed for reviewing paper due dates and dates of upcoming tests.

### SHARING HOUSEKEEPING TASKS

If you are living in a family situation, you need to delegate some tasks that were formerly yours to others in your household so that you can study the number of hours required for success in a nursing program. Your partner, if you have one, can help with household chores, run errands, and help with some of the tasks of child rearing. If adolescents are competent drivers, they can run errands and pick up and deliver smaller children for school or activities. (See further suggestions in Chapter 3.)

### WORK ADJUSTMENTS

Once you decide to begin a nursing program, check with your employer about the possibility of flexible hours to accommodate the need for extra study time before examinations and for hospital clinical rotation requirements. Many employers will adjust hours for nursing students. **To give yourself the best chance at success in the nursing**

TIME MAP
ACTIVITY

| TIME | SUNDAY | MONDAY | TUESDAY | WEDNESDAY | THURSDAY | FRIDAY | SATURDAY |
|---|---|---|---|---|---|---|---|
| 6 | | | | | | | |
| 7 | | Exercise | CLINICAL | CLINICAL | CLINICAL | Exercise | House work |
| 8 | Church or other | CLASS | | | | CLASS | yard work etc. |
| 9 | Family Activity | | | | | | Laundry & |
| 10 | | | | | | | Ironing etc. |
| 11 | Brunch | | | | | | |
| 12 | nap | Lunch | | | | Lunch | Prepare week's meals |
| 1 | Study | CLASS | | | | CLASS | |
| 2 | | | | | | | |
| 3 | | Errands | Errands | Errands | Errands | Errands | |
| 4 | | Time with Kids | Time with Kids | CLINICAL Prep | Time with Kids | Study | Exercise |
| 5 | Time with Family | CLINICAL Prep | Time with husband/wife | Pick up house | catch up time | | Study |
| 6 | Dinner | Dinner | Dinner | Dinner | Dinner | out for dinner | Dinner |
| 7 | Time with Family | Time with husband/wife | Study | Study | Study | Free time | movie etc. |
| 8 | Study | Study | | | | | |
| 9 | | | Bed | Bed | Bed | | |
| 10 | Bed | | | | | | |
| 11 | | | | | | | |
| 12 | | | | | | | |

**FIG. 1.2** Sample time map.

**program, try not to work more than 20 hours per week.** The recommendations of one college regarding work and number of units undertaken are as follows:

| | |
|---|---|
| 40 hours of work | Take only 6 units |
| 30 hours of work | Take only 9 units |
| 20 hours of work | Take only 12 units |
| 10 hours of work | Take only 15 units |
| 0 hours of work | Take 18 units |

Courtesy Allan Hancock College, Santa Maria, CA.

| TIME MAP<br>ACTIVITY | | | | | | | |
|---|---|---|---|---|---|---|---|
| TIME | SUNDAY | MONDAY | TUESDAY | WEDNESDAY | THURSDAY | FRIDAY | SATURDAY |
| 6 | | | | | | | |
| 7 | | | | | | | |
| 8 | | | | | | | |
| 9 | | | | | | | |
| 10 | | | | | | | |
| 11 | | | | | | | |
| 12 | | | | | | | |
| 1 | | | | | | | |
| 2 | | | | | | | |
| 3 | | | | | | | |
| 4 | | | | | | | |
| 5 | | | | | | | |
| 6 | | | | | | | |
| 7 | | | | | | | |
| 8 | | | | | | | |
| 9 | | | | | | | |
| 10 | | | | | | | |
| 11 | | | | | | | |
| 12 | | | | | | | |

**FIG. 1.3** Blank time map.

If, after the first few months of the program, you find you have extra time when you could work and you are doing well academically, then you may be able to increase the number of work hours. Work hours may have to be adjusted again later in the program as courses become more demanding. If your employer is not able to adjust your schedule, you may wish to find a job working as a technician or as a patient care assistant in the local hospital during your training period. Many hospitals offer tuition reimbursement and flexible schedules for nursing students. Some hospitals have scholarship funds available for employees as well.

Another temporary or part-time job is as a student assistant on campus. Most colleges have a part-time work program available for students, including department "gofers," part-time secretaries or receptionists, laboratory helpers, classroom aides, library helpers, and similar positions. These positions are limited and are awarded to the quickest applicants.

A third possibility for part-time employment may be available for those who have a previous college degree or who excel in certain subjects such as mathematics, English, or science. A tutor in the college learning or tutoring center can earn $10.00 or more per hour. The financial aid officer can provide information about grants and loans available and may also have scholarship information. The counseling center can assist you in your search for scholarship funds, as can both the school and local community librarians. Whatever your work schedule, enter your work hours in your calendar each week.

## Study Skills

The study of nursing requires a great deal of reading. Most nursing and science textbooks are written at a college reading level. If you doubt your reading efficiency, contact your counselor or academic advisor and arrange to have your reading skills evaluated. Once the evaluation is done and any problem areas have been identified, methods by which your reading efficiency can be improved will be suggested. The few hours spent learning how to read more efficiently can save you study time in the future. Many schools offer a college learning skills course, and some institutions target sections specifically to health occupation students. Such a class, which is usually only 1 credit hour, can be a great tool for success in the nursing program. Taking a medical terminology class prior to nursing school may help with reading comprehension.

Students in most nursing programs are expected to be proficient in how to access online materials and to use common software such as word processing and presentation programs. Many schools are using e-books for textbooks and are requiring the use of a laptop or iPad-type computer. Smartpens are available for taking notes and then uploading them for saving or printing. The pens are capable of recording audio lectures and then transferring the files to the computer as well.

Well-written professional nursing journal articles are invaluable resources. A bibliography or reference list for such articles is often included in your textbooks, the course outline, or the course syllabus. Check your college library's list of available journals in print or online (see Chapter 6). Ask the librarian to help if you are unfamiliar with accessing computerized databases. **Subscribing immediately to at least one of the major professional nursing journals when you enter nursing school is a time-saving idea.** Reading a journal each month will add considerably to your knowledge base in nursing. *Nursing 2017*, *Nursing Made Incredibly Easy!*, and the *American Journal of Nursing* are three journals most useful to nursing students. Most journals give students a discounted price. *Imprint* is the National Student Nurses Association journal and has articles that are directed particularly to students rather than practicing nurses.

Various websites have very helpful study aids such as flash card programs for learning drug names (see Chapter 6).

## LEARNING STYLES

Evaluating how you learn best is also helpful. Some people are visual learners, others are auditory learners, and some are tactile or kinesthetic learners, who learn best by doing. Most students have a predominant learning mode but use at least one of the other modes. The student learning center or counseling center, or the online tests listed in Chapter 6, can direct you in ways to evaluate your own learning style so that you can structure your studying around the best mode for you. If you are a visual learner, reading texts and articles and watching visual presentations via the computer or video are the best ways to spend your study time. Videos are easily found online for a variety of subjects (see Chapter 6). If you are an auditory learner, then recording lectures (after getting permission to do so), listening to supplementary CDs or MP3 lecture files, which are available at some schools, and perhaps reading and recording your texts for future listening are the best ways to study. A tactile learner needs to spend extra time in the skill and simulation lab or at home practicing the skills step by step, preferably with a peer watching. Computer-based instruction may also assist this type of learner by allowing some tactile interaction during the lesson. The actual performance of skills and patient care in the clinical setting is the other major mode of learning available for a tactile learner. Elsevier's Virtual Clinical Excursions, which are designed to complement your textbooks and incorporate visual, auditory, and kinesthetic learning, are available at your college bookstore or online from Elsevier Inc.

## TEXTBOOKS

Buy your required textbooks immediately in e-book or paper form, and put your name in any paper text. When studying, remember to check each possible text that might contain information required for the next day's lecture topics. Text information frequently changes in the health occupation field; therefore, relying on a friend's old textbooks is not a good idea. The required textbooks are essential to your success. If you cannot afford a textbook right now, visit the library to determine whether a copy is "on reserve." Read the library copy and make buying your own textbook a top priority.

### Reading

You will absorb more from your reading if you find a quiet place with few distractions. If you must read with activity going on around you, consider masking the noise and distraction by using a pair of foam earplugs (available at pharmacies) or headphones with soft music playing. Some students who are parents have found that it is best for them to go to bed at the same time as their children, get up in the middle of the night for a few hours to read and study, and then sleep a few more hours before the beginning of the day.

Read in an organized, consistent manner. **Look up unfamiliar words** in the glossary of the text or a dictionary as you encounter them, and jot down their meanings. The SQ4R study method (Box 1.3) is a popular plan for tackling reading and study assignments. Try it; if it does not suit your needs, check your college library and bookstore for study books containing other methods.

**Reading is the key to establishing the base of knowledge needed to function as a nurse.** If you can find time to read full chapters rather than just a few pages about a particular disease or problem, you will remember the information more easily and develop a fuller understanding of the body systems, how homeostasis is affected by diseases, and why particular nursing interventions are effective in a particular instance. From the beginning of nursing school, studying this way tends to make reading assignments less lengthy and makes the upper-level courses much easier, because you will already have read much of the material to be covered.

Nursing textbooks are large and heavy. If you have time to study at work, consider an e-reader (e.g., Kindle, iPad, Nook). Textbook companies have developed interactive texts for online use. If this is not an option, consider tearing out individual chapters in your paper textbook to take to work with you. Heavy books are difficult to carry, but single chapters are easily portable. (This may sound like heresy when you have been taught not to damage a book, but it is a practical solution.) Be certain to keep the chapters neatly filed for future review.

Students who have difficulty reading because of dyslexia or visual problems should contact the Braille Institute Library Services (1-800-272-4553; 741 North Vermont Avenue, Los Angeles, CA 90029). Students who qualify can receive recordings of various nursing textbooks as well as a tape or CD player to use with them. Students with other learning disabilities should contact the campus learning assistance center to see what testing and resources may be available.

## Using Ancillary Materials

Check out online resources designated for your textbooks or the CDs packaged with them, which usually contain a significant amount of good information. They

---

**BOX 1.3**

### SQ4R Study Method

| **S** Survey | **R** Read | **R** Record (Write) |
|---|---|---|
| **Q** Question | **R** Recite | **R** Review |

| | |
|---|---|
| Survey | Look over the chapter. Read all the headings, captions under photographs, and illustrations, charts, and graphs, plus the summary or last paragraph. This survey provides the core ideas in the chapter. |
| Question | Make a question out of each heading. Doing so arouses curiosity, focuses on the content, and brings to mind information you already know. |
| Read | Begin actively reading for an answer to the question. Read only one section and be certain you have answered the question before continuing. Highlight or underline the important points as you find them. |
| Recite | After finishing each section, look away from the book and, using your own words, recite the answer to your question. If you can do this, you know what is in the book. If you cannot, you need to reread the section and consider. Continue in this manner through the entire reading assignment. Write study notes for your syllabus objectives as you finish each section either by writing an answer to the objective or by making an outline for the items listed in the content column of the syllabus. |
| Record (Write) | Record the information in some fashion. Use a highlighter to mark directly on the specific information in the text, take notes, or use a combination of the two. It is important to read and understand the material first and then go back and record. |
| Review | When you have finished the assignment for the next lecture session, review your notes to understand the points and their relationships to one another. Check your memory by trying to answer each objective in the syllabus without looking at your notes. |

may include extras that would not fit into the text chapters, animations for various concepts or processes, audio pronunciation files, links to useful resources, and many other features. Checking for updates on the textbook's accompanying website is a good idea.

A helpful study guide or workbook may be available for your nursing text. If study guides are not *required*, check your bookstore or the Internet to see whether any are available for your texts. Many students find such resources useful learning tools.

## Taking Notes

Two types of notes should be taken: (1) preparatory notes taken before class and (2) class notes taken during a lecture or lab, which build on your preparatory notes. Preparation before class greatly enhances learning, because the material covered in class is not being encountered for the first time. **Repetition is essential to the retention of information.** Some e-book texts are interactive online, through Pageburst or similar software. The software allows you to add notes as you read, highlight material, and note questions. Familiarity with the topics to be covered in class allows you to follow the instructor's presentation by listening actively and adding to notes as needed. (When you attempt to take extensive notes during class, you might miss much of what the instructor is saying.)

Consult the course outline or syllabus to identify material that will be covered during each class. First, read the required selection in your textbook, underlining or highlighting key concepts in the text, tables, charts, and illustrations. Then create preparatory study notes by outlining the material covered in required reading or by writing out concise answers to the lecture or chapter objectives. When writing study notes, use an organizational method that allows for the addition of information during the lecture. As study notes are enhanced during the lecture, they become class notes.

Some instructors may provide Microsoft PowerPoint slides or other outlines for students to download and bring to class. This is a handy way to take organized notes in class. Two examples of study notes styles are offered in Fig. 1.4. Review each set of revised notes as soon as possible after class, review all notes for the week every weekend, and review all notes for material to be covered on an examination in the few days preceding the test.

Considering what would make a good examination question out of this material is also helpful. What questions would you ask if you were the instructor? Jot down your ideas. After the examination on this material, go back to see how many of these questions were on the test. While preparing for class, jot down any points that are unclear, but wait until the topic is covered to ask the questions, because the instructor will likely answer them or clarify the topic during class time.

Along with the required readings, the syllabus may also list other learning resources, such as related periodical articles from professional nursing journals, media presentations, and computer learning modules. Whenever material is difficult to understand or unclear, using one or two of these other resources can greatly improve comprehension and retention of the material.

## Recording Lectures

Some schools provide Microsoft PowerPoint with voice-over lectures on the school LMS. These are to be used before class time. The class time then provides other types of learning activities facilitated by the instructor. This is termed a "flipped classroom" method of teaching. Some schools still use the traditional lecture method for class time. If you have difficulty following a particular instructor's presentation or simply do not "get" all the information in a lecture, you may want to use an audio or video recorder during class (after obtaining the instructor's permission). It has often been said that the average student hears only 30% of what is said during a class period. Taking the time to listen to or watch the recordings and adding to your study notes as appropriate are necessary for the success of this type of study. You also can play audio recordings in the car when traveling to and from school and work or while preparing meals, doing yard work, ironing, or performing other household chores that lend themselves to listening while doing.

## Strengthening Computer Skills

Honing your computer skills will make you a more efficient and better organized student and nurse. You will be expected to use a unit computer to enter data about patient care when working or participating in clinical rotations and a word processing program such as Microsoft Word to create nursing care plans and written assignments. As you progress through your nursing courses, creating nursing care plans electronically can save a lot of repetitious writing. With files of saved care plans, you can cut and paste, individualizing the new plan for a particular patient.

Microsoft Excel is also a valuable program to learn and is used in almost any job. Microsoft PowerPoint will most likely be needed by students asked to make class presentations. This presentation software is used throughout the business world. E-mail is valuable for contacting fellow students and instructors and is also a useful way for a busy nursing student to stay in touch with friends. Skype or FaceTime can be used to work from home with other students.

The Internet is a wonderful source for information on medical and nursing topics, including patient teaching. Blogs, message boards, and chat rooms covering topics specific to nurses or nursing students can help you get answers to questions and provide a support group. You will be asked to do research, and the Internet has a wealth of information (and misinformation). Knowing how to evaluate the sites and information you find is essential (Box 1.4).

## Joining a Study Group

Depending on your learning style, you may find that joining a study group helps you better prepare for tests. The advantage of being in a study group is that you receive the benefit of the other members' viewpoints on topics and what is most important in the material to be covered on a test. Some study groups divide up the objectives of a unit, and each member prepares the answers to a certain number of the objectives. This method works well if each member does a thorough job. However, some students cannot simply read and memorize material; they retain the information better if they write it out themselves. **When looking for a study group, remember that studying with people who are more knowledgeable than you and earning as good or better grades is to your advantage.**

When working with a study group, complete the reading and prepare for a discussion before you meet. Discussing the material will round out your knowledge of the subject, and hearing about it again will reinforce it in your memory.

## Obtaining Tutoring

Check with the tutoring center, learning center, learning resources center, or college handbook to see whether tutoring service is available. Tutoring services are often free to students and are provided by a higher-level student who has

Study Notes                    Sept. 7, 2017
Unit One                       Chapter 8

| | |
|---|---|
| Objective 2: Describe the 5 Steps of the Nursing Process | – N.P. forms foundation for nsng practice. |
| Definition | – Used daily with patients and families. |
| Nursing Process: Series of planned steps & actions → meet needs. | – Process of using sequential steps to produce a desired result. – Systematic problem solving (Scientific method adapted to human beings ē unmet needs.) Lecture:   Circular process |
| 1. Assessment Collection and analysis of data | – Collect physical and psychosocial data via interview, observation, physical assessment, review of medical record, discussion with family or significant others). – Assessment is on-going Lecture: assess continuously; during bathing; effect of tx. Circular. Assess to evaluate. |
| 2. Nursing diagnosis | – Data analyzed to identify problem areas. – Clinical judgment about responses to actual or potential problems or life processes. – Nsg dx provides basis for selection of outcomes and then of interventions to assist person to meet outcomes. – Nsg dx s classified by North American Nursing Diagnosis Association |
| Fluid volume deficit | Lecture: NOT a medical dx. 1st part is the human response. |

**FIG. I.4** Two examples of study note styles.

Study Notes          Sept. 8, 2017
                          Chapter 8

Obj. 2    Describe the 5 steps of the nursing process

| | Lecture: |
|---|---|
| I. Nursing process | Circular, systematic |
| A. Foundation of practice | process similar to |
| B. Used daily | scientific method. |
| C. Sequential steps to- | Use with every patient. |
| ward desired result. | Core of professional |
| D. Systematic problem | nursing. Methodical |
| solving. | and orderly. |
| | |
| II. Assessment | Assessment is on-going. |
| A. Physical & psychosocial | Constantly assess - during |
| data gathered | bath & txs. Response to |
| 1) patient | meds. Assess in order to |
| 2) chart | evaluate. Use all senses. |
| 3) family / S.O. | History taking via inter- |
| B. Analysis of data | view. Physical assessment |
| | |
| III. Nursing diagnosis | Data analyzed to find |
| A. Identify human | problem areas. Requires |
| response | clinical judgment. |
| B. Related factors | North |
| C. Pertinent defining | American |
| characteristics | Nursing |
| D. Choose from NANDA | Diagnosis |
| list. | Association |
| | Not a medical dx. |
| | Basis for choosing |
| | interventions to alleviate |
| | human response. |

FIG. 1.4, cont'd

### Evaluating a Web Page    BOX 1.4

- Who wrote the page? What are the person's qualifications and associations? Can you contact him or her?
- What institution publishes this page? Check the domain of the document in the URL. Preferred domains are *.edu, .gov, .org,* and *.net.*
- When was the web page produced? Is it current and timely? Has it been updated since it was written?
- Is the information cited authentic? Can you verify it with other sources?
- What is the purpose of the web page?
- What is the point of view? What opinions are expressed by the author? Is bias evident? If so, what is it?
- Is the web page written objectively?
- Could the web page be a spoof or ironic?
- Are questions or reservations you have about the web page answered or satisfied?
- How up to date are the links (if they are provided)?

knowledge of the subject matter. Sometimes tutoring is available on a fee-for-service basis. The main point is to seek help as soon as you determine that you could use it.

### Taking an Online Course

When considering an online course, ask yourself whether you are a self-motivator and highly disciplined about schoolwork. Without face-to-face contact with an instructor, you will need to take the initiative in obtaining assignments, requesting clarification when questions arise, and completing required work. Before signing up for an online course, explore the course description and requirements, be certain that the computer you will use meets the minimum specifications and that you have the required software installed, and make sure the course will meet your needs (such as credit toward graduation, prerequisite credit for another course you will take later, or other requirements). If the class is offered by a different college from the one you are attending, be certain the credit will be transferable. Determine whether your level of computer competence is sufficient to get you through the course (Box 1.5).

Once you are enrolled, determine the instructor's expectations. If they are not clear, e-mail the instructor and ask for the specific expectations. Consider the expectations and how your own strengths fit with what is expected. Consider the challenges you will face in the course. Do you have the technical skills you will need? Become familiar with the software platform (e.g., Blackboard, WebCT, Canvas, E-College, etc.) through which the online course will be offered. If you are unfamiliar with the platform, work through the tutorial for it. If you have doubts about your academic research or computer skills, check with your librarian or the computer lab personnel. They can recommend materials and tutorials that may be helpful. Or check with the local community college. Many have free or inexpensive community and noncredit computer courses.

Time management is extremely important when you engage in distance learning. If the instructor sets virtual office hours, plan your study time around them to ensure that he or she will be available to answer questions quickly if they arise. If specific times for communication with fellow students or with the instructor are set, be online and available. Write these times into your daily time map.

Many online classes are organized into a series of modules. Set up files for each module, and keep everything together that pertains to each module. This method of organization will help you have everything ready when you work on a particular module. Accordion files are great for papers related to the module.

Be aware that Internet searches can be very time consuming. Schedule enough time to conduct your research, and start well ahead of the paper or project due date. Check the class bulletin board daily for postings from faculty or students.

Note that communication within an online course is slower than that in the classroom. Often a delay may occur between sending an e-mail question to the instructor and receiving an answer. When you do not understand something about an assignment or a reading, immediately seek clarification from the instructor. Be patient when waiting for an answer; do not send repeat e-mails with the same questions.

Often an online course will require you to work as part of a group on a project. Try to balance your interaction so that you do not end up doing more than your

---

**BOX 1.5**

## Computer Competency Checklist for Nursing Classes

You should know how to use the following software:

- Operating system (e.g., Microsoft Windows)
- Word processing program (e.g., Microsoft Word)
- Presentation program (e.g., Microsoft PowerPoint)
- Spreadsheet program (e.g., Microsoft Excel)

You should be able to:

- Gain access to an Internet service or service provider, preferably high speed.
- Enable a firewall.
- Use a virus protection program.
- Install software programs.
- Save a file of your work to your hard drive, a Google Drive, or a flash drive.
- Download and save files.
- Copy, cut, and paste sections of text within a document and between documents.
- Use an Internet search engine.
- Search for information and articles on a given subject.
- Burn a CD or DVD.
- Clear the cache or temporary Internet files in a web browser.

For accessing and handling e-mail, you should be able to:

- Set up an e-mail account with an Internet provider.
- Send, receive, and open e-mail messages.
- Open e-mail attachments.
- Reply to e-mail messages.
- Print e-mail messages.
- Save e-mail messages to folders.
- Attach files to e-mail messages.
- Delete e-mail messages.

share of the project. Keep communication open and timely among the group members so that progress on each part of the project will be evident. Because your grade depends on all members of the group finishing their portions, plan some extra time to help pick up the slack if someone does not come through with his or her part of the work.

Taking online classes can be beneficial because they are more time flexible than on-campus classes. You alone are responsible for scheduling when you will go online to do your class work. Some degree programs can be accomplished entirely by taking online courses (see Chapter 4).

## Doing Your Best on Tests

It is a good idea at the beginning of each week to scan your calendar for the next test date. The best way to decrease test anxiety is to study the material sufficiently and get a good night's sleep before the examination. Last-minute cramming does not work for most people. Because the National Council Licensure Examination (NCLEX) is a timed exam, nursing school tests have a time limit in which to complete answering the test questions. Testing may be done via computer in a designated computer room.

### PREPARATION

When organizing to study specifically for an examination, review the instructor's designation of the material to be covered on the particular test. Conduct this review at least 1 week before the test. Gather revised preparatory notes, and rewrite the data that you feel are most important (and likely to be included on the test) in a concise form. Include material from special sources, such as required presentations or articles. Review your concise test notes each night.

Divide the material into the same number of parts as number of days before the test, and systematically review your full notes at least once more. If time permits, you can go back and review what you have highlighted in your texts as well. If you belong to a study group, meet on the day before the examination and question one another on the objectives and what the group believes is the most important material as well as the material an instructor will most likely include in the examination. When preparing for an exam, be certain you know which type of testing will be used (computer or paper). Exams may use only generic drug names in questions because that is how the NCLEX exam questions are written. Nursing diagnoses (as listed by the North American Nursing Diagnosis Association [NANDA]) are not used on the NCLEX exam.

**Day before the examination.** Review the syllabus or course outline of the material to be covered on the test. Read the content column, as well as the objectives, and review anything you cannot immediately recall. Pay close attention to the vocabulary and terms.

**Night before the examination.** Get at least 7 hours of sleep. Eat a normal meal before going to school. If the test is late in the morning, take a high-power snack with you to eat 20 minutes before the examination. The brain works best when it has the glucose necessary for cellular function. Stay away from other nervous students before the test. Stop reviewing at least 30 minutes before the test. Take a walk, go to the library and read a magazine, listen to music, or do something else that is relaxing. Go to the test room a few minutes before class time so that you are not rushed in settling down in your seat. Tune out what others are saying. Crowd tension is contagious, so stay away from it.

### During the examination

*Paper tests.* You can enhance your chance of success during a test. The following are several suggestions for taking tests on paper:

- Note the number of questions and the total time allotted for the test to calculate the times at which you should be halfway and three-quarters finished with the test. Allow 5 to 10 minutes to check your work and your answer sheet. Look at the clock only every 10 minutes or so.
- Carefully read the preliminary instructions and check the whiteboard or screen at the front of the room for any changes, corrections, or additional instructions.
- Calm yourself by closing your eyes, putting down your pencil, and relaxing. Deep-breathe for a few minutes (or as needed, if you feel especially tense) to relax your body and to relieve tension.
- If you are allowed to write on the test materials, underline all pertinent data and circle key words in the question.
- Cover the answer options before reading the question on multiple choice tests. Read the question and think about what the answer(s) should be; then see whether such an answer is among the choices.
- For questions in which you need to "select all that apply," cover the answers while looking at the question stem and think about what fits. Then look at each of the choices and circle the number or letter of each choice that correctly fits with the question. For fill-in-the-blank exercises, choose the word or words that immediately come to mind. Some questions will ask you to identify a spot on an anatomic model where you would do something or where something occurs. Locate the landmarks on the model carefully before indicating the correct spot.
- Eliminate wrong choices by marking through the letters or numbers of those choices.
- After choosing an answer, go back and reread the question stem along with your chosen answer. Does it fit correctly? The choice that grammatically fits the stem and contains the correct information is the best choice.
- Do not read too much into the question or worry that it is a "trick." If you have nursing experience, ask yourself how a classmate who is inexperienced would answer this question from only the information provided in the textbooks or given in the lectures.
- If you do not understand the question or a word within the question, raise your hand and ask the instructor for clarification.
- Avoid choosing answers that use words such as *always*, *never*, *must*, *all*, and *none*. If you are confused about the question, read the choices, label them *true* or *false*, and choose the answer that is the odd one out (i.e., the one false one or the one true one). When a question is framed in the negative, such as "When assessing for pain, you should *not*...," the false option is the correct choice.
- Do not fret over any one question for too long. If you are having trouble, skip the question and go back to it when you have finished answering the other questions.

- If using a paper Scantron sheet, keep track of the correlating test question number. When you skip a question, be careful to also skip the corresponding space on the Scantron sheet.
- Check your Scantron sheet to ensure that every line has only one mark; two marks on any one line would throw all the remaining answers off track from the correct question numbers.
- Choose the best answer for questions asking for a single answer. More than one answer may be correct, but one answer may contain more information or more important information than another answer.
- When you are unsure, jot down what you know about the topic in the margin, or on permitted scratch paper, without looking at the answers. Then look at the answers and follow your best instinct.
- **Never erase and change an answer on a Scantron sheet** unless you have read the question or the answer incorrectly or remember a specific piece of information that has a bearing on the question. If you realize that you missed questions on previous tests because you erased and changed answers, cut the eraser off the end of the pencil you take to the examination. If you find you have read a question wrong and really need to erase, raise your hand and ask the instructor for an eraser. This technique has helped numerous students raise their test grades considerably.
- At the end of the test, reread the questions, making certain you understood each one correctly. Verify that the answer sheet is marked in the right location for each answer.

*Computer-based tests.* Many of these suggestions also are useful for tests administered via computer. In addition to these tips, it is wise to practice on the type of computer on which the test will be given. Maintaining focus without becoming distracted by people entering and leaving the room can be a challenge. Monitoring your time is very important. Most computer tests do not penalize you for guessing at an answer. With computer testing, usually you will not be able to skip questions and go back to answer them later. You will not be able to change an answer once you have progressed to the next question. Ask whether you will be allowed scratch paper in the computer testing room. Be certain you know the times the test is available for you to take in the testing location.

- When entering the test, click the link only once. It may take a while to load.
- Do not use the "back" button.
- Do not double click on an answer. A second click may be read as a second attempt to answer and may block further access to the test.
- Do not click "Submit," "Next," or "Save" more than once for each question.
- Do click on a blank area when using a mouse with a scroll wheel so that you don't accidentally change an answer when scrolling.
- Answer all the questions.
- If possible, review all your answers before you click "Submit" to enter your test answers at the end of the test. Click "Submit" only once.
- If the test is timed, you may be given a 1-minute warning before time is up. Be certain to click "Submit" before the time is up.
- Your test may be suspended if you click outside of the test itself. This is to prevent a quick Internet lookup of the answer. The proctor of the test will

verify that there was no cheating intent with the actions and authorize your continued testing. Be careful where you click your mouse.

## ALTERNATE-FORMAT QUESTIONS

You may find that questions on your examinations are not always multiple choice, in which a single option of four given is correct, and many are patterned after the types used on the NCLEX exam. Alternate-format questions include the following types; correct answers are given.

**Multiple response.** A patient is prescribed a low-fat diet. In counseling him or her about food choices, you would tell him or her to avoid (*select all that apply*):

1. Butter
2. Barbecued ribs
3. Grilled salmon
4. Caesar salad
5. Hamburgers
6. Whole milk
*Answer:* 1, 2, 5, 6

**Illustration/graphic.** The nurse is performing a physical examination on a patient. When listening to the heart, the nurse would place the stethoscope over the apex to count the apical pulse. Indicate on the diagram the location of the apex of the heart.

*Answer:* C

**Prioritization/sequencing.** When catheterizing a female patient, the nurse would use sterile technique. Place the steps of the catheterization procedure in the correct sequence.

1. Lubricate the catheter.
2. Don sterile gloves.
3. Cleanse the meatus.
4. Drape the genital area.
5. Locate the urinary meatus.
6. Insert the catheter.
*Answer:* 5, 4, 2, 3, 1, 6

**Completion/fill-in-the-blank.** A patient has an intravenous (IV) infusion ordered of D5 ½NS 1000 mL at 100 mL/hr. If the IV tubing will deliver 15 drops/mL, the IV should be set to deliver _____ drops per minute.
*Answer:* 25

**Chart/exhibition.** A patient had surgery yesterday with bleeding at the surgical site. Serial laboratory hemoglobin and hematocrit values have been measured as follows:

|            | 1600       | 2200       | 0800       | 1400       |
|------------|------------|------------|------------|------------|
| Hemoglobin | 10.8 mg/dL | 10.2 mg/dL | 10.2 mg/dL | 10.4 mg/dL |
| Hematocrit | 28%        | 26%        | 26%        | 27%        |

Assessment of the data reveals that:

1. Slow bleeding may be occurring.
2. Considerable blood loss occurred.
3. Red blood cell count has stabilized.
4. Red blood cell count shows hemodilution.

*Answer:* 3

**Other question types.** Other question types include true–false (mark true or false), short answer (write a brief answer), and matching (you are asked to choose the correct companions from column 2 that correlate with statements or items in column 1). NCLEX questions are also written in the traditional multiple-choice format (one correct answer from a choice of four).

## ESSAY EXAMINATIONS
- Divide the total testing time by the number of questions to be completed.
- Quickly outline the content of your answer before you begin writing.
- Answer the questions you know best first; doing so will help build your confidence.
- If you do not think you know the answer, take a little time to jot down everything you know about the topic and then try to formulate an answer.
- If you have absolutely no clue as to the answer to a question, try to think of something creative to write. Sometimes an instructor will give you a few points for creativity. Anything is better than a blank space on an essay examination.
- Reread each question and the answer you have written, making certain that it actually answers the question asked.
- Be certain your handwriting is legible.
- Pay attention to correct grammar, punctuation, and spelling.

## ACADEMIC HONESTY
Most colleges have an honesty policy or code, and nursing as a profession expects its members to be honest and ethical. Although learning may involve group activities, you must write papers or care plans alone and submit your own work. Colleges have software programs to detect plagiarism (work done by another but submitted as one's own). Cheating on tests—including copying from another's test paper or computer screen, acquiring answers from or giving answers to another person by

any means, discussing questions or topics from a test with another student yet to take the exams, and sneaking information into the testing area in any form—is often a cause for dismissal from a nursing program. Use of smartphones to take pictures of tests or having the phone out to use the calculator function and then doing a net search for a test question answer, are just some of the ways that students have found to cheat. Cell phones are not allowed in testing areas at most schools. You are expected to act ethically. Cheating does not prepare the student to pass the NCLEX exam.

If you think that an assignment is meant to be a group project and allows collaboration with others, verify that with the instructor. If you are writing a research paper, make sure you understand how to reference sources. Not giving credit to information sources is considered plagiarism. Cheating is a serious matter in nursing education because you must thoroughly know the information being taught to become a safe nurse. Once you become a registered or practical nurse, the lives of your patients are in your hands. **A mistake can mean serious injury or death.**

A saying in the human resources field is, "Past practice predicts future performance." If you cheat as a student, the prediction is that you may continue to do so as a nurse. Nurses have the privilege and responsibility of caring for patients when they are most vulnerable, and ethical practice is at the heart of nursing. Patients trust nurses and count on them to do what is in the best interest of the patient. Be worthy of that trust.

## TROUBLESHOOTING EXAMINATION PERFORMANCE

If you are not achieving the scores you would like or think you deserve, review the following questions to find ways in which you might improve your chance to score higher:

- How many hours per week are you spending in quality, uninterrupted study time?
- How well can you concentrate during each segment of your study time? Are you too tired to concentrate?
- How many hours are you working? How many credit hours are you taking? Do you have enough hours in the week to study adequately?
- Are you doing your reading before class? Are you reading whole chapters?
- Are you reading in each pertinent textbook (fundamentals of nursing, medical–surgical nursing, pediatric nursing, obstetric nursing, nutrition, psychiatric nursing, and pharmacology, among others)?
- How do you begin a unit of study? Do you review the pertinent anatomy and physiology before beginning the text readings if you do not remember the content?
- Do you study the objectives in the syllabus as you go, including the topics in the content column?
- Are you utilizing other assigned activities before class?
- Do you take study notes after you have first read the material but before the lecture in a format that allows you to add lecture notes to your study notes?
- Do you use a voice recorder in class? Do you review the recordings?
- Do you experience greater than normal test anxiety? Have you worked with a counselor for this anxiety? Have you regularly practiced suggested relaxation and confidence-building techniques?
- Do you review each day's lecture notes that night?

- Are you using effective test-taking techniques, as follows:
  - Becoming comfortable with the computer-type testing before the exam?
  - Underlining key words in the stem and choices (for paper tests)?
  - Eliminating wrong choices?
  - Checking to ensure that your chosen answer fits with the question stem and that it answers the question asked?
  - Using test time evenly?
  - Refraining from frequently erasing and changing answers?
- Do you have a regular study group or study partner? Are the others in the group doing well? (If not, study with someone who is!)
- Are you relying on reading in a review book to get you through instead of reading your texts?
- Are you relying on reading in a review book before tests instead of studying your own notes?

If you identify your problem areas and remedy them, your test scores will improve. Students often believe that they study a lot, but they study at home with constant interruptions to their concentration. Going to the neighborhood library to study is one option. Organizing to study during the day when roommates, partners, and children are out of the house, and then doing chores, shopping, laundry, and errands at night, is another alternative.

Problems at school should be remedied as soon as they are identified. Many students believe their school experiences will improve without taking any initiative to make certain that they do. Too often, students wait until they are in serious trouble with poor grades before changing their study habits or the number of hours they work. You have invested a lot in your education; guard that investment by giving yourself the best chance for success.

A psychological technique used to boost your test-taking confidence is to look into a mirror whenever you pass one and say out loud, "I know the material, and I'll do well on the test." Try it; many students have found that it works because it reduces "test anxiety."

## Taking the National Council Licensure Examination

During your final semester, you will receive information from your instructors on the mechanics of signing up to take the NCLEX exam, which is taken on a computer at a designated testing site. After you graduate from your nursing program and have met the educational requirements for licensure, your school will notify the state board of nursing that you have completed the required courses for licensure. You must submit an application for licensure to the state board of nursing, and then you will receive authorization that allows you to sit for the NCLEX-RN exam or NCLEX-PN exam, depending on which type of program (Registered Nurse or Practical Nurse) you have completed. The examinations are offered at sites across the United States. If you do not pass the test on the first attempt, you must wait 45 to 90 days (depending on the state you are in) before retaking it. The examination may be taken in any state, but licensure will be issued by the state in which you reside. Visit www.ncsbn.com to view the test plan, a variety of resources to help you prepare for the examination, and a list of states that have a reciprocity compact agreement for licensure (in which license is obtained in one state but education and passing the exam make one eligible to obtain a license in another state).

## Obtaining Licensure

After passing the NCLEX-PN exam or NCLEX-RN exam, you will receive notification from the board. Some states and licensing boards require an application/testing fee and then a separate fee for obtaining the actual license. Others require complete payment at the time of application and your license will be mailed after successful NCLEX exam completion.

# GETTING THE MOST FROM THE CLINICAL EXPERIENCE

2

## ■ APPROACHING THE CLINICAL EXPERIENCE

You may be assigned to various clinical facilities during the semester. Clinical locations include hospitals, long-term care facilities, home health agencies, community clinics, psychiatric outpatient clinics, day care centers, rehabilitation facilities, and school clinics. At some of these facilities you may be an observer rather than a care provider. Your instructor will clarify how you should prepare for the type of clinical facility to which you are assigned.

It is normal to be concerned and apprehensive about your first contact with a patient. Be assured that you will not be required to do more for the patient than your nursing course has prepared you to do. Remember that there is always a staff nurse assigned to the patient as well. It is usual for the student to prepare at school for the skills to be performed in the clinical setting and to be evaluated on critical skills by an instructor. Only then are you expected to apply your skills with real patients. Critical skills are those in which accuracy is of vital importance to the patient's treatment (e.g., taking vital signs) or those that are invasive and have a potential for injury to the patient (e.g., giving an injection, inserting a urinary catheter).

If you are entering the room to take vital signs, be certain you have all your equipment with you including appropriate documentation resources—paper, handheld electronic device, or in-room computer. Some electronic blood pressure (BP) devices have a built-in printer; make sure it has paper.

Most students fear hurting the patient. The best way to prevent harm is to be as prepared as possible for the clinical patient assignment and to refuse to perform tasks for which instruction and verification of the correct technique by an instructor have not yet occurred. Tell the nurse in charge of the patient that you may not perform the skill or care involved if you have not covered it in school.

### Preparing for Clinical Patient Care

At some schools, instructors assign patients to the students; other schools require that each student choose patients for the clinical assignment. Either way, you will receive some pertinent information ahead of time. Before you see the patient, you will know the patient's diagnosis, what treatments are scheduled, any tests the patient may have that day, the names of the patient's medications, and the patient's age and sex. Conduct a quick review of each patient's chart when obtaining your information (Table 2.1). In addition, ask to see the patient care card, Kardex plan, or electronic patient care sheets. These provide directions for everything the nurse should be doing for the patient. Look for the nursing care plan or the "problem"

| TABLE **2.1** Quick Chart Review | |
|---|---|
| **Item** | **Information** |
| Admission information | Marital status, age, insurance coverage, occupation, significant others, religion, location of home |
| Physician's orders | Tests ordered, medications, intravenous solutions, treatments to be done, code status (admitting day up to today) |
| Physician's history and physical (H & P) | Overview of total health status and summary of current and physical health problems; allergies |
| Physician's progress notes | Clues to future tests and orders; status of notes problems |
| Medication reconciliation | Medications and supplements taken at home |
| Patient medical history | Allergies; height and weight; prosthetic devices such as hearing aids, glasses, or contact lenses; previous health problems and hospitalizations; previous surgery; and so forth |
| Laboratory reports | Tests that have been completed, results, and any abnormal values |
| Other test results | Findings that are abnormal (read the conclusions); pathology reports tell whether patient has cancer |
| Medication administration record (MAR) | Medications ordered; how often patient is taking as-needed (PRN) medications and what they are |
| Consultations | Conclusions of other members of the health care team |
| Nursing assessment/notes | Vital signs, intake and output, blood administered, assessment data |
| Nursing care plan, collaborative care plan, care pathway, or "needs" list | Lists the problems or nursing diagnoses, with goals and care interventions to be done |
| Operative report | Conclusion tells what was done; abnormalities found and problems encountered; amount of blood loss |

list in the chart; both will give you some ideas about the patient's nursing problems. Before selecting your assignment, check with the nurse in charge to ensure that you know which patients other students have already selected.

Preparing for clinical patient care involves reading about the disease process or problem and noting the following:

- Causes and contributing (etiologic) factors
- Usual signs and symptoms of the disorder
- Common treatment for the disorder, including medications
- Common nursing problems or nursing diagnoses the patient is likely to have
- Expected outcomes
- Psychosocial ramifications

If you are not assigned a specific patient before your clinical experience, find out which unit you will be assigned to and determine the types of patients usually cared for on that unit. Then read about those types of patients. For example, if you are assigned to an orthopedic unit, you should read about fractures, back problems, and hip and knee replacements. When you are assigned to a general surgical unit, review preoperative and postoperative care, dressing changes, nasogastric suction, and care of wound suction devices and catheters, among others. Your textbooks will give you clues about the information you will need for the type of hospital unit in which you will be working. An Internet search can usually provide information on the disease or condition a patient has and the appropriate care. Search by subject or enter a medical website such as those listed in Chapter 6. If you do not have your own computer or a smartphone, use one available at your school or the public library.

## Reviewing Skills for Patient Care

Review information about the treatments to be provided, such as dressing changes, maintaining traction, hot or cold applications, and intravenous (IV) therapy. You should review each treatment even if it is not a task you are capable of doing. Clinical learning takes place when you are prepared and observe an experienced nurse perform the skill. Of course, as each nursing course progresses, you will be prepared to perform more of the skills. Instructors generally require that the student review a skill just before performing it in the clinical area.

When on the nursing unit, you can look up the skill or treatment in the procedure manual kept on the floor or in the computer. Each nursing unit should have a manual available to staff that provides the specific steps and protocol for performing each nursing procedure. To be within safe, legal boundaries, each nurse should perform the designated procedure in the manner described. It is up to the student to seek experience in performing skills. Choose patients for your assignment who require some skills you can perform. Mention to the staff nurse that, when your assigned work is done, you would like to perform other tasks for which you are prepared. Be specific about what you are looking for, such as injection, catheterization, or IV therapy experience.

## Looking Up Medications

**From clinical day 1, you should look up each medication your assigned patients are receiving.** Learn the generic name as well as the most common brand name. Although students do not usually administer medications during the first weeks of the first nursing course, the best way to learn about the thousands of medications in use is to attach a patient situation to each. Even if you are not giving the medication, you will be expected to watch for possible side effects of various drugs. **You are legally liable if you cause harm to a patient from a medication error you committed.**

### DRUG TEXT APP OR HANDBOOK

If you have a pharmacology text, look up and review each patient's medication(s). If you do not have such a text, you may wish to purchase a drug reference written especially for nurses or an application (app) for your smartphone or tablet. Many such books are available on the market, and your school bookstore probably stocks a variety of handbooks. Information you want includes the following:

- Classification of the drug (e.g., antibiotic, antihypertensive)
- What the medication is supposed to do for the patient (i.e., its action in understandable terms)
- Usual dosage and route of administration
- Potential serious adverse effects
- Common side effects

- Drug interactions
- Patient data (e.g., BP prior to BP meds, potassium level for potassium supplements)
- Special nursing implications (e.g., whether the medication needs to be given with food or an hour after meals, whether sunlight should be avoided)

Most electronic health record (EHR) software has a built-in drug reference that is useful for a quick check when giving meds. As a student, medication information will be remembered longer if it is read, noted in writing, and reviewed several times. Electronic resources are helpful but do not replace learning.

To reduce your fear of making a medication error, review the "Safety Guidelines to Prevent Medication Errors" in Chapter 5. If you understand how a drug works, you will be able to determine the possible side effects and nursing implications. When you are well prepared for each clinical experience, you will be less anxious and will be able to function in the clinical setting more efficiently. And you will have less fear of hurting a patient and will learn more.

## GUIDELINES FOR USE OF MOBILE DEVICES

Know which devices are acceptable (or not) in the clinical agency. Many facilities provide a mobile telephone to unit nurses for intrafacility communication. Electronic devices are usually regulated because of the potential for interference with medical equipment, breaches in confidentiality, and lack of professionalism (Brant et al, 2016). Make sure to know the policy of the clinical facility. Some allow use of personal devices and some restrict use of *all* devices. If a handheld device is used in the clinical setting, make sure to sanitize it on a regular basis and never lay it down on a surface in a patient room. Use good hand hygiene and be mindful of what the device has touched so contamination can be avoided.

If a personal device is permissible, make sure never to take pictures in the clinical setting. Even if you are not taking pictures of a patient, protected information may inadvertently be photographed. Confidentiality breaches are usually grounds for dismissal from the nursing program, and the hospital can be fined for your actions if they violate federal law. Use the device ONLY for what is intended. If you are allowed to use a device to look up drug and clinical information, it is not appropriate to check social media sites while on the unit. Be responsible and accountable in complying with facility and nursing program policies regarding electronic devices.

## MOBILE DEVICES AND SOFTWARE

Some schools of nursing are recommending a portable handheld device such as a smartphone, pocket PC, or tablet for use in the clinical setting. Make sure to verify the policy of the facility for use of personal devices. Some facilities do not allow student access to the EHR, and alternate charting may be done using these devices. Software programs that are very helpful in clinicals include the following:

- Nursing diagnosis/care plan manual
- Guide to clinical procedures
- English–Spanish (or other language) medical word and phrase program
- Guide to evidence-based practice
- Manual of diseases and disorders with specific information on assessments, nursing diagnoses, and management of commonly seen disorders
- Handbook of laboratory and diagnostic tests with nursing implications

- Drug guide
- Medical dictionary
- Calculator

# ■ NURSING CARE PLANS

After instruction on the nursing process, you probably will be required to create a written nursing care plan or concept care map for each clinical day. Some schools require a certain number of problem statements or nursing diagnoses to be worked out; others want a complete care plan for each patient. From the data gathering you did for your assignment, you will have the patient's medical diagnoses, diagnostic test data, some history, and nursing diagnoses or problems that were listed in the facility care plan. Analyze your data and determine your own nursing diagnoses or list of patient problems as you were taught in your fundamentals of nursing course.

Practical nursing (licensed practical nurse/licensed vocational nurse [LPN/LVN]) students may be given the patient's problem statements/nursing diagnoses and asked to construct a plan based on the identified problems. Each problem statement/nursing diagnosis must be correlated with supporting data. Determine appropriate goals or outcome criteria for each diagnosis. Ask yourself whether the expected outcome you have written is measurable; in other words, will you be able to tell from evaluation data whether it has been met? Is the goal obtainable? Is it something that can actually be accomplished? "SMART" goals should be used— Specific, Measurable, Attainable, Realistic, and Time-specific. When writing nursing care plans or designing concept care maps, you must pull together information you have learned from anatomy and physiology, microbiology, and psychology courses as well as your nursing courses, and must apply this information to a particular situation. Your fundamentals of nursing text plus the text for the specific clinical area to which you are assigned (e.g., obstetrics, medical-surgical, pediatrics, psychiatric) will provide information for usual problems and nursing actions for patients with the medical diagnosis or problems your patients have.

## Nursing Diagnoses

Your school may not use nursing diagnoses as defined by the North American Nursing Diagnosis Association (NANDA) because many health facilities do not use them. Some nursing schools may still use them. Many nursing care plan books generalize nursing diagnoses and actions for a particular disorder. Your school bookstore may stock several of these books. Choose one that is easy to understand and that is as close as possible to the format your school uses. Be aware, though, that you still must individualize the care plans for your patients. Many of these books have the care plans on a CD or website that you can individualize for your patients. Read through the plan listed and ask yourself whether each item applies to your specific patient before including it in your own nursing care plan. Nursing care planning is a thinking process, not simply a copying process. The whole idea is to systematically devise a plan to meet a specific patient's basic needs. It is best to look at patients holistically, including their psychosocial and physical needs. One way to check yourself when writing care plans is to see whether you have covered all areas of basic need. Box 2.1 offers a checklist for choosing nursing diagnoses/patient problems using the acronym RN'S HOPE to ensure that you have considered all areas. **Two problems that students often overlook are limitations in self-care and lack of knowledge about the disease or its treatment.**

BOX 2.1

## Choosing Problem Statements/Nursing Diagnoses

Once you have analyzed your assessment data and selected the most obvious problems for your patient's nursing care plan, you should review each area of possible need to ensure that you have not missed an important area. One way to conduct this review is to keep in mind the acronym RN'S HOPE, which covers all areas of basic needs:

**R** Rest and activity
**N** Nutrition
**S** Safety
**H** Hygiene
**O** Oxygenation
**P** Psychosocial
**E** Elimination and education

   Examples of problem statements grouped for each area of basic need include the following:

**REST AND ACTIVITY**
- Altered activity tolerance
- Altered physical mobility
- Fatigue
- Disrupted sleep pattern
- Pain: acute or chronic

**NUTRITION**
- Altered nutrition
- Altered self-care ability: feeding
- Potential for constipation
- Potential for unstable blood glucose level
- Altered swallowing ability
- Fluid volume: deficient or excess
- Nausea
- Potential for electrolyte imbalance

**SAFETY**
- Acute confusion
- Potential for contamination
- Altered sensory perception
- Potential for injury
- Altered physical mobility
- Potential for infection
- Altered skin integrity
- Potential for impaired skin integrity
- Potential for peripheral neurovascular dysfunction
- Altered verbal communication
- Hyperthermia
- Hypothermia
- Potential for falls
- Altered memory ability
- Wandering

**HYGIENE**
- Inadequate health management

## Choosing Problem Statements/Nursing Diagnoses (cont'd)

- Inability for self-care: toileting
- Inability for self-care: dressing
- Inability for self-care: bathing
- Potential for altered oral mucous membrane

### OXYGENATION

- Alteration in airway clearance
- Potential for aspiration
- Potential for altered tissue perfusion
- Altered breathing pattern
- Altered gas exchange
- Altered peripheral tissue perfusion
- Altered cardiac output

### PSYCHOSOCIAL

- Limited coping ability
- Altered decision making ability
- Dysfunctional impulse control
- Altered family functioning
- Fear
- Anxiety
- Altered body image
- Inadequate health maintenance
- Decreased ability for home maintenance
- Post-trauma distress
- Moral struggle
- Altered role performance
- Decreased self-esteem
- Spiritual disconnection
- Potential for social isolation
- Stress overload

### ELIMINATION AND EDUCATION

- Constipation
- Altered urinary function
- Urinary incontinence
- Diarrhea
- Bowel incontinence
- Altered self-care ability: toileting
- Fluid volume excess
- Altered sexual function
- Insufficient knowledge

*Some schools may use NANDA nursing diagnoses rather than problem statements.* Remember that many nursing actions are used to prevent problems, and in this event these actions are grouped under a "risk for" nursing diagnosis. The three areas students most often overlook are altered self-care, insufficient knowledge, and the major reason the patient is in the hospital, such as fractured hip (altered physical mobility) or myocardial infarction (altered cardiac output). In addition, **each medication to be administered and each procedure to be performed should fit under some problem statement on the care plan as an intervention.**

Each instructor views nursing care plans a bit differently, even within a particular school of nursing. Get to know what your instructor wants and how things should be worded in general. Ask to see an example of a nursing care plan that the instructor thinks is very good.

## Interventions

Read your textbooks for ideas about actions that are appropriate to meet the patient's needs for each problem. For example, if the problem is potential infection related to poor nutritional status, then, in addition to monitoring for signs of infection—such as increased temperature; increased white blood cell count; redness, pain, and swelling of the wound; and purulent drainage—you would include actions to improve nutritional status. Such actions would be to increase protein and vitamin C intake and encourage a well-balanced diet with sufficient fluids and calories to maintain a positive nutritional balance. Of course, using good hand hygiene and aseptic techniques for dressing changes and using Standard Precautions are included as well. Actions must be individualized for each patient; actions for the patient who has diabetes might be a little different from those for a patient who does not.

Evidence-based practice should be the major focus for choosing interventions for your care plan or care map. (See Chapter 6 for a list of suggested websites for searching the evidence.)

## Rationales

Many programs require a scientific rationale or principle for each action listed on your care plan. What is desired is a science-based reason to explain how the action works. An example for interventions included in the sample nursing care plan in Fig. 2.1 is the following:

Intervention: Discourage intake of foods high in caffeine.
Rationale: The chemical caffeine causes blood vessels to constrict, increasing
     blood pressure.

A sample concept map or care map, sometimes used in place of a full nursing care plan, is illustrated in Fig. 2.2.

## EVALUATION

The evaluation section of the nursing process cannot be completed until you carry out your plan of care during clinical hours. After you have cared for the patient, go back and review your preliminary plan. Evaluate whether the plan accomplished the goal or at least made progress toward it. Some of the problem statements/nursing diagnoses you listed may not be pertinent, and you may have discovered other problems and concerns that are more important to the patient. Delete actions that are ineffective, and devise new ones to help meet your stated expected outcomes. Usually the care plan does not have to be recopied or redone; you just add to it, perhaps in a different color (paper or computer) to show what has been changed and updated.

## PATHOPHYSIOLOGY STATEMENT

Some programs also require a pathophysiology statement concerning the patient's medical diagnosis or problem. For beginning courses, a simple explanation of the

Getting the Most from
the Clinical Experience

## Sample Nursing Care Plan

Selected problem statements/nursing diagnoses, goals/expected outcomes, nursing interventions, and evaluations for a patient with hypertension

**Situation:** 53-year-old male with a blood pressure of 170/100 found during routine screening of all employees at a local plant. A visit to the hypertension clinic reveals that he is hypertensive, is 75 pounds overweight, smokes two packs of cigarettes a day, and eats snacks during the day and in the evening while watching television. The physician prescribes a low-sodium diet and a mild antihypertensive. During her interview with the patient, the nurse notes that he does not understand the nature of his illness, how his lifestyle is related to hypertension, and the purpose of the low-sodium diet and the expected action of the medication.

| Problem Statement/Nursing Diagnosis | Goals/Expected Outcomes | Nursing Interventions | Evaluation |
|---|---|---|---|
| **Altered peripheral tissue perfusion** *as evidenced by* BP, 172/102; P, 96; feet cool and pale; pedal pulses, 1+; capillary refill > 4s. | Patient will maintain adequate tissue perfusion as evidenced by: 1. BP within normal limits at end of 3 weeks. 2. Pulse returns to normal range within 4 weeks. 3. Skin of feet warm and dry within 4 weeks. 4. Capillary refill time less than 3 sec within 4 weeks. Patient will quit smoking within 1 month. | Teach to take antihypertensive as ordered; and monitor BP bid. Assess skin and peripheral pulses each visit. Discourage smoking; encourage him to quit smoking. Discourage intake of foods high in caffeine. Maintain sodium restrictions. Have patient weigh himself daily and keep record. | BP, 156/96; P, 86; skin on feet pale and cool; smoked only five cigarettes today; weight down 2 lbs. Continue plan. |
| **Altered nutrition, excess calorie intake** *as evidenced by* weight, 285 lbs; height, 6 ft; consumes lots of junk food between meals; no daily exercise program; watches a lot of television. | Patient will lose 2 lbs within 2 months. Consultation with dietitian within 2 weeks. Patient will maintain 2-lb/wk weight loss until normal weight of 210 lbs is attained. Patient will have developed daily exercise plan within 2 weeks. | Explain need to lose excess weight; encourage him to participate in weight loss plan. Assist with development of daily exercise plan. Ask for dietary consult. | Weight, 283 lbs; is considering options for daily exercise plan. |

**FIG. 2.1**  Sample nursing care plan. *BP,* Blood pressure; *P,* pulse.

Sample Nursing Care Plan—cont'd

| Nursing Diagnosis | Goals/Expected Outcomes | Nursing Interventions | Evaluation |
|---|---|---|---|
| **Insufficient knowledge related to management of hypertension** *as evidenced by* lack of ability to take own blood pressure; unsure about new antihypertensive medications; unfamiliar with low-sodium diet; unaware of need for regular exercise to control weight and blood pressure; complaints of cost of going to the doctor. | Patient will demonstrate correct technique for taking own blood pressure within 1 week of teaching. Patient will explain action of antihypertensive medication and possible side effects 1 week after teaching session. Patient will describe effects of exercise on cardiovascular system after teaching session. Patient will state which foods are high in sodium when given a list from which to choose foods after teaching session. Before discharge patient will give three reasons why continued follow-up is necessary for patients with hypertension. | Develop teaching plan covering the following points: 1. How to take own blood pressure. 2. Action and side effects of antihypertensive medication. 3. Beneficial effects of exercise program on cardiovascular system. 4. How sodium increases water retention and elevates blood pressure. 5. Foods to avoid that contain excess sodium. 6. Potential complications of uncontrolled blood pressure and reasons for physician examination to detect beginning complications. | First teaching session completed; verbalizes action and three side effects of antihypertensive medication; can pick foods high in sodium from a list. Continue teaching and plan. Progressing toward outcomes. |
| **Inadequate health management** *as evidenced by* lack of desire to quit smoking and that he doesn't really need to do so because all of his friends smoke. | Patient will verbalize how smoking affects the blood vessels 3 days after teaching session. Patient will verbalize desire to quit smoking within 1 month. Patient will institute a "no smoking" program within 1 month. | Teach how nicotine constricts the blood vessels, elevating blood pressure and decreasing blood flow to the periphery of the body. Encourage patient to quit smoking. Obtain American Heart Association, American Lung Association, and American Cancer Society materials regarding the dangers of smoking. Familiarize the patient with available community "Quit Smoking" programs. Encourage him to join support group for those who are quitting smoking. | Discussed effect of smoking on vessels; gave patient AHA materials to read; encouraged him to quit smoking; scheduled another session tomorrow. Continue plan. |

**FIG. 2.1,** cont'd

**The Patient with a Fractured Femur**

**FIG. 2.2** Sample concept map or care map. *ADLs,* Activities of daily living; *LT,* long term; *ST,* short term.

diagnosis, including the physiological changes the disease or disorder is causing and the signs and symptoms expected, is usually all that is necessary. **If the patient is undergoing or has undergone surgery, complete the pathophysiology statement on the disorder that necessitated the surgery.** Include the type of surgical procedure performed and the physiological changes that the patient has experienced.

In more advanced courses you should consider the course of the disease or disorder and the prognosis if there is no intervention. Determine what the potential complications of the disorder may be, and discuss the effect of the problem on the patient's basic needs. Box 2.2 provides two examples of pathophysiology statements. Fig. 2.3 illustrates a pathophysiology concept map.

Writing pathophysiology statements helps you understand what is going on physiologically in the patient and how the condition is causing interference with the patient's ability to provide for his or her own basic needs. That is where you put

BOX 2.2

# Examples of Pathophysiology Statements

A pathophysiology statement usually consists of the etiology of the disease or disorder, the usual signs and symptoms in comparison with the individual patient's signs and symptoms, the usual treatment, and potential complications.

## EXAMPLE 1: CHOLELITHIASIS

Cholelithiasis is the presence of gallstones in the biliary system. The stones may be located in the gallbladder, the common duct, or the hepatic ducts of the liver. The stones may consist of cholesterol, pigments (mainly unconjugated bilirubin), or a combination of these substances with calcium carbonate, phosphate, or bile salts. Gallstones occur more frequently in women, and the incidence increases with age. This patient has the following risk factors: obesity, diabetes mellitus.

Usual signs and symptoms include pain, often in the upper right quadrant; jaundice; nausea and vomiting; bloating and indigestion; and fatty food intolerance. This patient has upper midline pain radiating to the right shoulder blade, nausea, and an intolerance to fatty foods.

Treatment consists of surgically removing the stones or breaking up the stones with lithotripsy or by chemical dissolution. This patient underwent laparoscopic cholecystectomy.

Complications include residual stones in a duct causing blockage, infection from the surgical procedure, and internal bleeding from surgery.

## EXAMPLE 2: MYOCARDIAL INFARCTION

Atherosclerosis → coronary thrombosis (or embolus) → occlusion of artery → myocardial tissue perfusion → impaired muscle function → ↓ cardiac output*

Potential complications include the following:

- Necrosis of tissue
- Dysrhythmia
- Heart failure
- Death

* Can be illustrated in the form of a concept map.

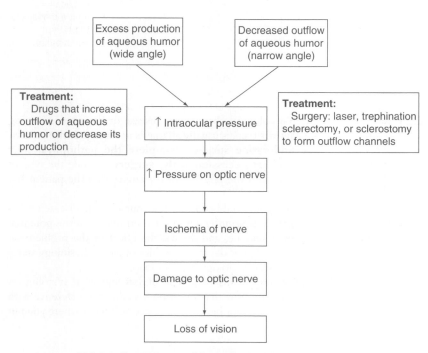

**FIG. 2.3** Concept map of the pathophysiology of glaucoma.

your nursing actions to work—you assist the patient in meeting basic needs when he or she is unable to do so. You can attempt to prevent complications that would extend the illness or delay the surgical recovery. Your understanding of the clinical condition helps you determine what assessments and monitoring should be done to evaluate the effectiveness of the treatment plan and to be able to identify the onset of complications early in the process.

Together, your chart review, preparatory reading, pathophysiology statement, and construction of the preliminary nursing care plan provide you with most of the data you need to care adequately for your patient. You will add information from a shift report to help determine what care your patient will need that day.

## Listening to the Shift Report

When listening to the morning or evening report (Box 2.3), you should write down pertinent information about your patients and all nursing care to be performed on your student activity organization sheet (Fig. 2.4). If you did not understand something, ask the nurse in charge about it. Verify with the staff nurse who is assigned to your patient your understanding of what you are responsible for in the care of the patient, and **state those tasks that are beyond your skill level.** Make certain that

---

### Information to Obtain During Report                    BOX **2.3**

Much of the following information should be available at the time of report on a report sheet, Kardex, or other communication tool. Some things will not be discussed in report unless there is a problem. If a patient is on a regular diet and has no difficulty eating or with nausea, it will not be part of a verbal report but the type of diet will be listed on the sheet. Items in italics below are topics that should be included in the verbal report.

- Room number and bed designation, age and gender of patient
- Date of admission and physician(s)
- Reason for admission and current diagnoses *Is the patient getting better?*
- Date of current surgery or delivery and type:
  - Vaginal or C-section
  - Gravida
  - Para
- Mental status if other than alert and oriented
- Surgery or tests scheduled for next 24 hours *If any prep, consent, or teaching is already done or is needed*
- Vital signs schedule if other than routine *Any abnormalities in readings*
- Specific assessments on a schedule
- Diet *How the patient is tolerating diet*
- Finger-stick glucose *Any insulin coverage given*
- Tubes: *Type and amount of output*
  - NG
  - Foley
  - Drains
- Oxygenation (if pertinent to patient condition)
  - $O_2$ sat goal
  - Type of $O_2$
- IV location, type, when inserted *Any problems with the site*

Continued

## Information to Obtain During Report (cont'd)

- Equipment:
  - Fetal monitor *What has been identified*
  - SCD
  - CPM *How the patient is tolerating, when it was last off*
  - Traction/type *How the patient is tolerating*
  - Telemetry *Cardiac rhythm and any abnormalities*
  - Other
- Treatments:
  - Dressing changes *Condition of dressing and wound*
  - TCDB
  - Spirometer *What the target is for the patient; how the patient is tolerating*
  - Heat/cold
- Activity: *How the patient is tolerating*
  - PT consults
  - Self-care ability
- Pain level:
  - Pain management *Frequency of medications*
  - PCA *Type of medication and settings*
- Medication changes *Why and how is the patient responding?*
- Problems
- Concerns/need for order changes
- Needed teaching
- Psychosocial status
- Patient–family dynamics
- Anticipated discharge date

*CPM*, Continuous passive motion; *C-section*, cesarean section; *IV*, intravenous; *NG*, nasogastric; *TCDB*, turn, cough, and deep breathe; *PT*, physical therapy; *PCA*, patient-controlled analgesia; *SCD*, sequential compression device.

the staff nurse understands that you do not perform tasks or assessments beyond your skill level. **This clarification is your responsibility.** Nurses work with students from different schools and different course levels. Unless you state differently, the nurse may assume you are doing everything that needs to be done for the patient, and vital assessments and treatments may go undone. Although you are not responsible to personally do everything for the patient, you are responsible to see that all necessary care is done.

### Preparing for Patient Teaching

From the patient assignment information and your reading about the disease process and nursing care, you will have an idea of the areas in which patient teaching may be required. If the patient will be having a diagnostic test, read about the test and especially note the pretest and post-test nursing care. If appropriate, ask to accompany the patient for the test to develop firsthand knowledge of what the patient experiences. This information will give you an edge in answering patient questions and help you know what to expect during your time of care. Having this information also helps with clinical time organization.

Other areas in which teaching may be necessary include self-care tasks such as cast care, dressing changes at home, diabetic self-care, medication administration, preoperative teaching, and any other health care–related task the patient and family

Student Activity Organization Sheet

| Patient/Room | 0730 | 0800 | 0900 | 1000 | 1100 | 1200 | 1300 | 1400 | 1500 |
|---|---|---|---|---|---|---|---|---|---|
| J.D. 521 | V.S.<br>Focused Assess | Meds<br>Shower<br>0830 Δ dressing | Meds | Full Assessment | Chart | V.S.<br>Glucometer | Pre-op teaching | Meds<br>Chart | |
| R.S. 523[1] | V.S. | Feed<br>Full Assessment<br>Turn | Meds | Bathe &<br>Bed<br>Turn<br>Chart | Chart | Feed<br>Turn<br>V.S. | Meds | Chart<br>Turn<br>Chart | |
| BW. 523[2] | V.S.<br>Focused Assess<br>√IV | Meds<br>√IV | Full Assessment<br>√IV | √IV | Assist<br>bath<br>Bed<br>√IV | √IV | Meds<br>√IV | √IV | √IV |
| Patient/Room | | | | | | | | | |
| Other activities | | | | 10-minute break | | Lunch break | | I&O if 8-hour shifts | Give report |

**FIG. 2.4** Sample student activity organization sheet. *I&O,* Intake and output; *IV,* intravenous; *Meds,* medications; *Pre-op,* preoperative; *V.S.,* vital signs.

---

### Checklist for Discharge Teaching

BOX **2.4**

Instructions must be given to each patient and family or significant other before discharge. Provide written instructions whenever possible in addition to verbal instructions, and cover the following topics:

- Medications—Name, dosage, times to be taken, side effects, special instructions
- Diet—What to eat, foods to avoid
- Activity—Exercise, rest, lifting, stair climbing, driving, resumption of sexual activity; special instructions for use of crutches, cane, walker
- Breathing exercises—Schedule for deep breathing and coughing or for incentive spirometry
- Wound care—How to cleanse the wound and change the dressing, signs and symptoms to report; management of any drains
- Bathing—Type of bath or shower permitted
- Next contact with the physician—When to call for appointment or time of appointment
- Signs and symptoms to report—Report temperature higher than 100.1° F, increase in pain, nausea and vomiting; particular instructions for individual patient
- Special instructions—Any specific points necessary for proper self-care

---

will be performing at home. Teaching for home care should begin as early as possible in the patient's hospital stay. In the acute care setting patients stay for 4 to 5 days on average, with many staying less time. That leaves very little time for effective patient teaching. Useful materials for patient teaching can be found in your textbooks and on the Internet. Search by topic or visit one of the medical websites listed in Chapter 6. Useful diagrams or sets of instructions for self-care are sometimes available to give the patient. Most facilities have online materials that can be customized and printed for the patient to use while hospitalized and to take home.

Every patient must receive discharge teaching and instructions before being released from the hospital. Find out what the hospital requires and what materials are available in print or on the in-house TV system or intranet. The topics covered are essentially the same for each patient, but the amount of instruction and the variations in care necessary at home depend on the patient's diagnosis or problem. Box 2.4 presents a checklist for discharge teaching so that you will be prepared if your patient is discharged on your clinical day.

### Organizing Your Workday

Regardless of the number of patients you are taking care of, organize your workday. Decide what you are going to do at which times according to the priority of the tasks. The shift report and chart review have given you data about the times that various things must be done. Vital signs are usually taken at 8:00 AM (0800), 12:00 PM (noon) (1200), 6:00 PM (1800), and 12:00 PM (midnight) (0000). Hospitals use the 24-hour clock, also referred to as "military time" (as shown in parentheses; see inside front cover). Get used to recognizing the 24-hour designations; it is the time signature for all hospital functions. If treatments are scheduled twice a day (bid) or three times a day (tid), you will have some flexibility in deciding when you wish them to be done (whether you can do them or not—consult your staff nurse). Consider whether the patient will be having physical therapy or special tests. Will the patient be off the unit or busy with the therapist? Ask the staff nurse. Plan what

**PATIENT CARE WORKSHEET**

| PATIENT | ROOM # | DIAGNOSIS | V/S | DIET | I&O | ACTIVITY | MISC. |
|---------|--------|-----------|-----|------|-----|----------|-------|
|  |  |  |  |  |  |  |  |
|  |  |  |  |  |  |  |  |
|  |  |  |  |  |  |  |  |
|  |  |  |  |  |  |  |  |
|  |  |  |  |  |  |  |  |
|  |  |  |  |  |  |  |  |
|  |  |  |  |  |  |  |  |

**FIG. 2.5** Patient care worksheet. *I&O,* Intake and output; *V/S,* vital signs.

time you will bathe the patient, make the bed, and do your more complete physical assessment. When will you do the dressing change or have the patient ambulate? Plan the time for turning, deep breathing, supervised use of incentive spirometer, and coughing. Should the patient be up in a chair for meals? Provide periods when the patient can rest. If you have several patients, plan your tasks in rotation so no one is neglected. Each patient should be seen at least every hour during the day shift. Initially, you will probably be assigned to only one patient. By the end of the first semester, you should be caring for at least two patients.

Fig. 2.4 provides a sample student activity organization sheet. A well-done shift activity organization sheet provides a good guide by which to do your charting. At the end of each clinical day, review your activity organization sheet to determine whether your plan worked. If it did not, think about what to change before you use the form again. Fig. 2.5 is a sample of a patient care worksheet similar to that used by many nurses to jot down information during report.

## Complying with HIPAA Requirements

Federal privacy regulations came into effect in April 2003 with the overall Health Insurance Portability and Accountability Act (HIPAA). The rules govern how

BOX **2.5**

## Patient Rights and Provider Responsibilities Covered by the Health Insurance Portability and Accountability Act (HIPAA)

- Consent—Written consent must contain a clause that says the patient agrees to allow the provider to use and disclose his or her information for treatment, payment, and health care operations. A notice must be attached to the consent form.
- Notice—The provider's obligations are outlined regarding the privacy of the patient's health care information. It includes the six patient rights and the responsibilities of the provider. It details how the patient information will be protected and a process for filing a complaint if the patient believes privacy rights have been violated.
- Access—The patient has the right to inspect and copy his or her medical record.
- Amendment—A patient has the right to amend his or her record for the purpose of accuracy.
- Accounting for disclosures—Providers are held accountable for how a patient's medical information is handled. Tracking any disclosures of information that were not related to treatment, payment, or health care operations, or that were not authorized by the patient, must occur.
- Restriction of disclosure—The patient can request that the provider restrict the use and disclosure of his or her information. The provider does not, however, have to grant the request.

Adapted from Williams P: *Fundamental concepts and skills for nursing,* ed 5, St. Louis, 2018, Saunders.

patient information is conveyed, stored, and shared. Box 2.5 presents a synopsis of the major points. **You must not discuss anything about your patients or clients with anyone who is not directly involved in their care.** Refrain from talking about your patients with others assigned to the same unit in the elevators or the cafeteria, where you may be overheard. **If you are documenting via computer, do not leave the screen unattended while a patient record is viewable.** Refrain from writing patient names on your written work; use only initials. When performing patient teaching or answering questions, keep your voice low and provide as much privacy as possible. Do not allow anyone not directly involved in the patient's care to view the medical record. HIPAA gives patients the right to correct erroneous information in their records and the right to the information in the record. Follow the agency's procedure if the patient requests to see the medical record. In many instances the medical record is available to the patient only after discharge.

Cell phones are not to be used within the public areas of the hospital while you are on duty. It is not professional to carry on personal conversations during your clinical hours. Patients should never be discussed with others, including family, colleagues on other units, or staff in the elevators. Never take pictures of anything on the patient unit with your cell phone camera. If you have a home emergency, ask permission to leave the floor and go to a private place to return the call. Otherwise, wait until you are off duty and outside the premises or in a private area.

HIPAA law extends to any comments about a patient on the Internet. **You must not blog or comment about a patient in any way on social networking sites or your own blog, even if names are not used.** Do not discuss anything to do with a patient outside of the clinical unit or with anyone other than your clinical instructor.

## Reviewing Basic Communication

Knowledge of the basic principles of therapeutic communication is essential for establishing rapport and trust and using specific techniques to facilitate interaction. Practice using therapeutic techniques whenever you can. Listen beyond the words, and look for the feelings the patient is trying to convey.

### NONVERBAL CUES (WHAT TO WATCH FOR)

Watch for nonverbal communication in body posture, facial expression, gestures, hand movements, and foot swinging, among others. Ask yourself whether the nonverbal clues fit the words.

### VERBAL CUES (WHAT TO LISTEN FOR)

Express interest in and encouragement for what the patient is saying. Nod your head, maintain eye contact, and say "uh-huh" or "mmm." Lean slightly toward the patient. Use reflection for the feeling you sense behind the words, and ask for feedback from the patient as to whether what you perceive is correct. For example, a statement such as "I sense that you are unsure about what to do" allows the patient to validate or correct your impression.

### USING SILENCE

Use silence appropriately; it gives the patient time to gather thoughts and formulate a response. Summarizing the highlights and main ideas of the interaction gives the patient a chance to correct any misperceptions and to know clearly what has been relayed to the nurse.

### ELICITING A RESPONSE

Use open-ended questions that will elicit more than a one- or two-word answer. Asking "who," "what," "where," or "how" requires the patient to elaborate when answering. Use "why" questions with caution and rarely; they tend to make the patient feel defensive. Table 2.2 provides examples of therapeutic communication techniques and barriers to communication.

| TABLE 2.2 | Quick Therapeutic Communication Review | |
|---|---|---|
| Technique | Example | Rationale |
| **Therapeutic Communication Techniques** | | |
| General leads | "Go on." "I see." "Uh-huh." "Please continue." | Encourage patient to continue or elaborate |
| Open-ended questions or statements | "Tell me more about that feeling." "I'd like to hear more about ..." "How did it start?" | Encourage patient to elaborate rather than answer in one or two words |
| Offering self | "I'm here to listen." "Can I help in some way?" | Shows caring, concern, and readiness to help |
| Restatement | *Patient:* "I tossed and turned last night." "You feel like you were awake all night?" | Restates in different words what the patient has said and encourages further communication on that topic |

Continued

**Quick Therapeutic Communication Review (cont'd)**

| Technique | Example | Rationale |
|---|---|---|
| Reflection | *Patient:* "I'm so scared about the surgery; anesthesia terrifies me." "Can you tell me how anesthesia terrifies you?" | Reflecting same words back to patient. It also encourages further verbalization of feelings |
| Seeking clarification | *Patient:* "Seeing my little girl come visit me was so hard. I'm so upset." "Your daughter upset you?" | Seeks clarification if the little girl upset the patient or her leaving was the upsetting factor. Helps the patient clarify unclear thoughts or ideas |
| Focusing | "Do you have any questions about your chemotherapy?" "Let's look at your options." | Asking a goal-directed question helps the patient focus on key concerns |
| Encouraging elaboration | "Tell me what that felt like." "I need more information about that." "Tell me more about the experience." | Helps the patient describe more fully the concern or problem under discussion |
| Giving information | "The test results take at least 48 hours to return to us." "You will get a preoperative injection that will make you sleepy before you are taken into the operating room." | Informs the patient of information relevant to specific health care or situation |
| Looking at alternatives | "Have you thought about …?" "You might want to think about …" "Would this be an option?" | Helps patients see options and consider alternatives to make their own decisions about health care |
| Silence | *Patient:* "I don't know if I should have chemotherapy, radiation, or both." [Nurse remains silent] | Maintaining silence and sitting attentively but quietly allows patients time to gather their thoughts and sort them out |
| Summarizing | "You've identified your alternatives pretty clearly." "You are aware of the important signs and symptoms to report to your physician; plan to call to make an appointment next week." | Sums up the important points of an interaction |

**Blocks to Effective Communication**

| Technique | Example | Rationale |
|---|---|---|
| Changing the subject | *Patient:* "I'm so worried about my husband." "It is time for your bath now." | Deprives the patient of the chance to verbalize concerns |
| Giving false reassurance | "I'm sure it will turn out fine." "You don't need to worry." | Negates the patient's feelings and may give false hope, which, if things turn out differently, can destroy trust in the nurse |
| Judgmental response | "I don't think that was a good thing for you to do considering you have diabetes." | Implies that the patient must take on the nurse's values and is demeaning to the patient |

**Quick Therapeutic Communication Review (cont'd)**

| Technique | Example | Rationale |
|---|---|---|
| Defensive response | *Patient:* "My doctor never seems to know what is going on." "Dr. Smith is a very good doctor; he's here every day." | Nurse responds by defending the doctor. Prevents patients from feeling that they are free to express their feelings |
| Asking probing questions | "Why were you there at that hour?" "What did you intend to prove?" | Pries into the patient's motives and therefore invades privacy |
| Using clichés | "Cheer up, you'll be home soon." "This won't hurt for long." "You have a long life ahead of you." | Negates the patient's individual situation; stereotypes the patient. This type of response sounds flippant and prevents the building of trust between patient and nurse |
| Giving advice | "If I were you, I would ..." "I think you should ..." "Why don't you ...?" | Tends to be controlling and diminishes patients' responsibility for taking charge of their own health |
| Inattentive listening | Turning your back when the patient is sharing feelings or pertinent information; showing impatience with body language (i.e., tapping your foot or having your hand on the door to go out). | Indicates that the patient is not important, that the nurse is bored, or that what is being said does not matter |

Adapted from Williams P: *Fundamental concepts and skills for nursing*, ed 5, St. Louis, 2018, Saunders.

## HELPING THE PATIENT CHOOSE

Assist the patient to solve the problem. Do not give advice or opinions. Let the patient choose alternatives that appeal to him or her for solution of the problem. Help explore what the alternatives might be, and then let the patient choose what is best.

## Approaching the Patient

Plan your first approach to the patient. If you are entering to take vital signs, be certain that you have all your equipment with you, including a piece of paper on which to write the results. Respect the patient's privacy and knock before entering the room. One way to approach the patient is, "Good morning, my name is _____, and I will be working with _____ (staff nurse) as your student nurse today." If it is the late shift, simply substitute "hello" for "good morning." Inquire how the patient slept last night or how the day has gone so far. Listen attentively. Express appropriate reactions or nod gently. Explain what you are going to do, and then do it.

To interview the patient and gather the data you need for your assessment, explain that you have looked at the chart but that your instructor requires that you ask a lot of questions that have probably already been asked by the physician or other nurses. Explain that a part of your learning experience is to interview the patient yourself. When you have gathered the data you need, perform a beginning quick assessment following the guidelines in Box 2.6. This type of quick assessment

# Quick Head-to-Toe Assessment

BOX **2.6**

At the beginning of each shift, each patient should be assessed quickly. This assessment is often performed along with the vital signs. Assessments may also be done according to body systems.

## INITIAL OBSERVATION
- Is the patient breathing?
- Skin color
- Appearance
- Affect
- How is the patient feeling?

## HEAD
- Level of consciousness
- Appearance of eyes
- Ability to communicate
- Mentation status

## VITAL SIGNS
- Temperature
- Pulse rate; rhythm
- Respiration rate, pattern, and depth
- Oxygen saturation
- Blood pressure (compare with previous readings)

## PAIN LEVEL
- Use pain scale
- Determine location*

## ABDOMEN
- Shape
- Soft or hard
- Bowel sounds
- Appetite
- Last bowel movement
- Voiding status

## EXTREMITIES
- Normal movement
- Skin turgor and temperature
- Peripheral pulses
- Edema

## TUBES AND EQUIPMENT PRESENT
- Intravenous catheter: condition of site, fluid in progress, rate, additives
- Oxygen cannula: liter flow rate
- Pulse oximeter: intact probe, readings
- Nasogastric tube: suction setting, amount and character of drainage
- Urinary catheter: character and quantity of drainage
- Dressings: location, drains in place, wound suction devices, character and amount of wound drainage
- Traction: correct weight, body alignment, weights hanging free
- External fixator, pin location appearance, drainage
- Other equipment (CPM, SCDs, etc.)

## HEART AND LUNG ASSESSMENT
For patients with current or potential heart or lung problems, auscultation of the heart and lungs should be performed on the initial assessment. For patients without these problems, auscultation can be performed later in the shift.

*CPM,* Continuous passive motion; *SCDs,* sequential compression devices.
* Pain is assessed whenever vital signs are measured.

should be done within the first hour of your shift. You will be able to gather additional history and data about the patient as you interact with him or her throughout the shift. An in-depth physical assessment can be performed a little bit at a time during the shift, but a baseline assessment of the patient's primary problem(s) needs to be done at the time of your quick assessment so that you can identify changes if they occur.

Assisting with the bath provides a prime opportunity to develop rapport with the patient and to focus the conversation on his or her concerns. You can also conduct a significant amount of physical assessment at that time—skin condition, range of motion of joints, ability to follow instructions, and level of alertness and cognition, among others. Your priority is to keep the interaction focused on the patient and not on yourself. A fine balance exists between the social interaction the patient needs and the professional interaction you need.

## Learning from the Staff

The unit secretary or clerk can be an ally if you are kind and friendly; you want this person "on your side." Address the person by name, and be considerate. Do not interrupt his or her work if you can help it.

The charge nurse is ultimately responsible for the patients on the unit. This is the person to consult about patient assignments and problems. However, it is the staff nurse you will work with most closely. This nurse may be a registered nurse (RN) or an LPN/LVN. In either case, this person can teach you a lot. Remember that nurses have different personalities, strengths, and weaknesses just like everyone else. You will work with some very experienced nurses and some who are fairly recently out of school themselves. Some staff nurses like working with students more than others. Which type of person you have on any given day is not predetermined. If the staff nurse likes to teach, use his or her expertise to the maximum. If you are finished with your patient care, ask whether you can shadow the staff nurse while he or she cares for other patients.

If you are working with a nurse who makes it obvious that a student is an inconvenience, simply stay out of the way, keep the nurse posted on assessments and tasks completed for your patient, and use your instructor as your primary resource for the day. The nurse may just be having a bad day or may have a patient who is not doing well, which may make him or her worried and preoccupied. It is not usually a personal reaction toward you. Talk with your instructor about your feelings. Try to remember the times when you have not wanted a younger sibling around or were angry with family members for one reason or another. Follow the correct lines of communication; however, do not skip giving this nurse information that is needed about the patient. Remember to "report off" to the nurse at the end of your shift.

When other health care professionals work with the patient, try to learn about what they are doing. Ask the respiratory therapist to show you more about the oxygen device in use. Watch the speech therapist work with the patient; then you can help the patient practice the exercises. Listen when the dietitian provides diet counseling, and you will be able to reinforce the teaching with the patient. Go with the physician when he or she visits the patient. Listen to what the physician tells the patient, because many times after the physician leaves the patient will ask for clarification of what was said. Ask any questions of the physician after you leave the room.

## Staying in the Good Graces of Your Instructor

Find out exactly what your instructor expects of you in the clinical area, and question any instructions you do not understand. Most instructors expect the following:

- Thorough preparation for the clinical and lab experiences
- Written work that is legible and neat
- A professional, clean, crisp appearance and demeanor in compliance with school and agency dress code
- A friendly, quiet, professional demeanor
- Sufficient sleep before the clinical experience
- Promptness for clinical and conference
- Active participation in clinical conference
- A quick, organized report on your patients when approached during the shift
- Cooperative, team attitude with the staff
- Attentiveness to patient needs
- Appropriate and complete documentation
- Attentive listening and attention to instructions
- Seeking of skill experiences
- Taking responsibility for your own learning
- To find you in the patients' rooms when you are not charting, rather than sitting at the nurses' station
- Asking questions when you do not know how to do something or whether it is permissible for you to do it
- To be notified immediately if something untoward happens or if a mistake is made

Recall that the role of the instructor is to correct and instruct you; do not take every comment made by the instructor as a personal attack. Some are better at gently correcting than others. Your instructor is there to prevent you from harming a patient. The instructor is your safety net. If you happen to have an instructor whom you cannot seem to please, make an appointment to talk about it. Ask what you can do to make the situation better. Tell him or her how you are feeling; your instructor is there to help you.

## Preventing Errors and Harm to Patients

Always be attuned to patient safety factors. When the bed is raised, keep side rails up when you are not at the bedside. Remember to lower the bed when you have finished working with the patient and lower side rails per agency protocol. Always turn around when leaving the room and survey it. Does the patient have the call bell within reach? Are the items needed within reach?

Do not attempt to move an incapacitated patient by yourself unless you are certain you can manage the correct technique for a safe transfer. Get help—it is not worth the risk of hurting the patient or yourself. You, in turn, can help others on the unit to move their patients. Learn to use the patient lifts that are available.

If you are told that a tube or IV cannula is to be removed from your patient, always check the chart and **read the actual order before taking the tube out**. Re-inserting a tube or IV cannula that was withdrawn in error is not a pleasant experience, and it subjects the patient to unnecessary discomfort and risk of infection.

Follow the accepted *six rights* (see Chapter 5), *five responsibilities*, and *three checks* method for administering medications. Perform the first two medication checks in the medication room or at the cart. Take the medication administration record (MAR) to the patient along with the medications, and check/scan the identification armband immediately on approaching the patient. Ask the patient to state his or her name and birth date while verifying the information with the chart. Then check/scan each medication appropriately with the MAR a third time just before administering it to the patient. Document that the purpose of the medication and possible side effects were explained to the patient. Document that the medication has been given only after the patient has taken it. Immediately report abnormalities in vital signs to the staff nurse assigned to the patient. Discuss anything else you find unusual or of concern about the patient. Talk with your instructor about your concerns as well. It is better to have a concern checked out than to assume it is probably nothing to worry about.

Always report to the nurse when you leave the unit for a meal so that someone else will check on your patients while you are gone. Be certain your charting is caught up before you leave the floor.

### Reviewing Documentation

There are many different systems of documentation within clinical facilities today (Box 2.7). You should receive information about the particular system used in your clinical facility and some guidelines for charting. If you do not receive this information, ask for it. There should be a charting or documentation manual available on the unit or on the facility intranet. You may be documenting on the computer or using a documentation simulation system required by your school such as SIMChart. Your documentation of patient care in the facility EHR or paper chart is a legal record; it must be comprehensible, objective, complete, and legible if handwritten.

---

## Types of Documentation for Nurse's Notes                    BOX **2.7**

**SOURCE-ORIENTED OR NARRATIVE CHARTING**
Phrases and sentences are written out without any standardized structure, content, or form. Care given is documented in chronologic order. Assessments usually follow a body systems format. Portions of lines are not left blank.

**Example**
4/10/12 0830 States has an increasing ache at a 6 on a scale of 1 to 10 in the right
    hip. Began after being in the chair for breakfast. T. 98.4, P 82, R 16, BP 138/88.
    Unrelieved by position change.
0845 Vicodin tab × 1 PO
0940 States pain has decreased to a 3.

R. Sims, RN

**PROBLEM-ORIENTED MEDICAL RECORD CHARTING FOR PROGRESS NOTES**
All health care personnel chart on the same forms and sequentially as care is given. A SOAP format is used (**S**—subjective information, **O**—objective data, **A**—assessment data/impression, **P**—plan). Some agencies modify to a SOAPIE or SOAPIER format that adds **I**—implementation, **E**—evaluation, and/or **R**—revision.

Continued

## Types of Documentation for Nurse's Notes (cont'd)

**Example**

4/12/12 1000 Pain, chronic

S  "The pain in my lower back is getting worse. It is a 7 on a scale of 1 to 10. It increased after I walked in the hall."

O  Forehead furrowed. Legs pulled up toward body. P 88, R 18.

A  Increased lumbar back pain.

P  Medicate with oxycodone as ordered.

T. Munoz, RN

### PIE CHARTING

PIE charting is an offshoot of SOAP charting. After designating the problem in one column, the note is formatted as **P**—problem identification, **I**—interventions, and **E**—evaluation.

**Example**

4/13/12 1420

P  States pain has increased with inspiration and it hurts to deep breathe or cough.

I  Medicated with albuterol inhaler 2 puffs at 1430.

E  Pain eased by 1445. Able to complete use of incentive spirometer and to cough.

J. Porter, RN

### FOCUS CHARTING

Focus charting is directed at a nursing diagnosis, a patient problem, a concern, a sign, a symptom, or an event. There are three components to the note: **D**—data, **A**—action, and **R**—response. (**E** may be used instead of **R** and stands for evaluation.)

**Example**

4/14/12 1300 Impaired skin integrity right heel

D  Heel red with 2-cm abrasion at base.

A  Cleansed with sterile saline and applied Tegaderm. Elevated heel off of bed.

R  2200 redness subsiding.

T. Moran, RN

### CHARTING BY EXCEPTION

Charting by exception assumes that all standards of practice are carried out and met with a normal or expected response unless otherwise documented. Documentation is done on a set of flow sheets, and a longhand note is written only when the standardized statement on the form is not met.

### ELECTRONIC CHARTING

Electronic charting is done by scrolling through a variety of screens on the computer and indicating care given and essential data about the patient. Mobile workstations or handheld devices are used so that documentation can be done at the bedside in real time. Medication administration documentation includes use of bar code scanning for patient identification and drugs and their doses. There are several software systems in use for electronic charting.

It is best to organize before beginning to enter your nurse's notes. Chart from an outline format or chart from the data on your student activity organization sheet. Much information is recorded on flow sheets in the chart or electronic record, such as the graphic record for vital signs, intake and output (I&O) sheet, daily activity or daily assessment form, IV flow sheet, and MAR. However, in any documentation system, any abnormal findings must be recorded in the nurse's notes along with a description of the action taken to correct the problem. Electronic systems have a mechanism for free texting nursing notes for checklist items that need further documentation.

Most hospitals require that a nurse document data for each nursing diagnosis, problem, or "need" in the patient's chart or electronic record at least once every 24 hours. For the nursing student, assessment data and actions should be recorded for each problem dealt with during the shift. General guidelines are listed in Box 2.8.

If the hospital or clinical site is using an EHR system and the facility allows computer documentation by students, training will be provided. When training is complete, you will receive a password to access the system. Carefully read over what you have entered before pressing the Enter key or "OK." Your log-on name and password constitute your electronic signature. Log off the computer properly. **Never leave a computer without logging off.** Never enter data when someone else is logged on, and do not let anyone else use the computer when you are logged on. Keep the computer screen out of the view of visitors to protect the patient's privacy.

### Giving a Report

When you leave your assigned unit for the day, you must "report off" to each nurse in charge of the patients assigned to you. If a nurse is on break when you are about to leave, "report off" to the charge nurse and make certain it is understood that you have not given your report to the primary nurse for the patient. Box 2.9 provides an outline of the information you should supply to each primary nurse for your assigned patients.

## ■ DEVELOPING PROFESSIONALISM

Nursing as a profession is striving to establish and maintain a professional image in the eyes of the public. The image you project as a nursing student and then as a nurse contributes to the overall public image of nursing. For this reason, nursing instructors will be teaching you about professionalism; they also will be evaluating you on your professional behavior. Image has three basic components: (1) appearance, (2) behavior, and (3) verbalization.

### Appearance

Appearance includes clothes and grooming. Besides wearing the required uniform components, their cleanliness and neatness contribute to your image. Underwear should not be visible beneath a uniform, slips should not show beneath the skirt hem, buttons should not be missing, pocket corners should not be torn loose, hose should not have runs, shoes should be polished, shoelaces should be clean, and shoes should have quiet soles. Depending on agency and school policy, visible tattoos and facial piercings may not be permitted.

Personal grooming of hair, beard, nails, and skin integrates with attire to project the visual image. The professionally groomed image includes keeping skin clean; wearing an effective, nonperfumed deodorant; and keeping nails clean and trimmed. Long nails make patients uneasy and are known to harbor bacteria. Infection control guidelines require that nail length be no more than one-quarter inch. Nail extenders or false nails are not to be worn because they carry bacteria. For men, the face should be clean-shaven or the beard neatly trimmed. For women, makeup should be minimal and low key, and nail polish should be

## Documentation (Charting) Guidelines

BOX **2.8**

Think of your charting as a camera that takes the patient's picture.

**ORGANIZE YOUR THOUGHTS**
- What have I seen that relates to this problem?
- What have I done about it?
- What do I plan to do about it?
- How has my patient responded to what has been done?
- Do I have the right chart?

**BUILD YOUR PLANNING ON YOUR**
- Initial assessment and further findings
- Identification of the patient's problems
- Patient care

**GENERAL GUIDELINES FOR PAPER CHARTING**
1. Chart neatly, legibly, and in black ink.
2. Be brief, concise, accurate, and complete.
3. Use good grammar, correct spelling, correct punctuation, and proper terminology.
4. Note the time of each entry; in addition, include the month, day, and year at the beginning of the shift charting.
5. Use a new line for each "new" (timed) entry. Draw an ink line through the extra space on a line you are charting if you have not used the entire line.
6. DO NOT ERASE. Draw a single line through an error; write "incorrect," "error," or "mistaken entry" over it; and sign your initials and the date (check agency procedure). Where room is available in the margin or above the corrected error, note the reason for it (e.g., wrong chart).
7. Never chart in advance of doing something; in particular, do not chart medications before they are administered.
8. Include your signature and student designation (e.g., SN). Use your first initial and last name with that designation.
9. Leave out the word *patient*. If the meaning of the entry is ambiguous, use the patient's name.
10. Use only those abbreviations accepted in your agency. (See the documentation guidelines for the agency.)
11. Retain recopied pages in the back of the chart (i.e., corrected graphic record).
12. Check on the correct format for charts in your clinical facility.
13. Use flow sheets whenever possible—do not duplicate the information in the nurse's notes.
14. Use easily defined terms (e.g., "ate 75% of meal" rather than "ate well").
15. Rather than "tolerated well," state outcome: tolerated without pain, without nausea, or without complaint. (*Well* means different things to different people.)
16. At the end of your shift, check through your charts to ensure that notes are complete, that entries on flow sheets are finished, and that each note is signed. Check through medication administration records (MARs) for your assigned patients, and make certain that no medication has been overlooked and that you have initialed every medication you administered.

**CONTENTS TO INCLUDE FOR ELECTRONIC OR NON-ELECTRONIC DOCUMENTATION**
*Physical care:* type of bath, back care, skin care and assessment, mouth care, hair care, perineal care, position changes (most data go on flow sheets)

## Documentation (Charting) Guidelines (cont'd)

*Intake:* diet, amount eaten as a percentage, fluids (oral, nasogastric [NG], intravenous [IV]); IV site condition, type of fluid, equipment changed, complaints (use activity sheet, intake and output [I&O] sheet, IV flow sheet)

*Output:* emesis, bowel movement, wound drainage, tube drainage, urine, vaginal flow, perspiration; include amounts and appearance (I&O sheet, nurse's notes)

*Treatments:* time, type, duration, appearance of area treated, special equipment, specifics of procedure (how it is done), patient response; if left unit, time left and by which conveyance, time returned

*Tests:* laboratory specimens drawn, cultures, disposition of specimens; radiographs, sonograms, endoscopies, patient reaction; if left unit, time left, by which conveyance, time returned

*Dressings:* appearance of incision or wound, smell, presence of drainage and appearance, how redressed and by whom

*Activity:* time; ambulation and distance; exercises performed, including leg and breathing postoperatively; range of motion (ROM) performed; physical therapy; condition of pressure points; repositioning and for how long; and patient response to each

*Oxygen:* time applied or amount changed, method of administration, safety precautions

*Medications:* time, amount, route, response, any adverse reaction or side effects, omission or delay, evidence of expected action (as needed [PRN] and immediate [STAT] doses are charted on the MAR and in the nurse's notes)

*Sleep:* day or night; amount, interruptions; patient comments

*Mental state (be objective):* mood, level of consciousness, general behavior

*Preoperative preparation:* teaching, physical preparation, time, and by whom; patient questions

*Special conditions:* traction; cast; special equipment, time applied, amount of weight, condition of patient, circulation checks and findings, skin condition, smell

*Vital signs:* temperature, pulse, respirations, blood pressure

*Physician's visits:* examinations, treatments

*Visitors:* who, how long, patient reaction

*Feelings:* what patient states regarding feelings, complaints, concerns

*Physical assessment:* what you see, hear, smell, and feel; auscultation of lungs, heart, bowel sounds; palpation of abdomen and pulses; inspection of skin; assessment of problem area in depth

*Safety factors:* side rails up or down, replaced after working with patient; warnings; security devices in place

clear or light in color and not be chipped. For both genders, hair should be secured so that it does not swing over the patient while you are performing care and should not have unnatural colors. Hair contains bacteria that can fall on the patient. Jewelry also harbors microorganisms; only a plain wedding band and watch should be worn in the clinical areas. Other types of rings and bracelets may injure the patient's skin while the nurse is giving direct care; furthermore, you may lose a stone or break a bracelet if it catches on something. A good guideline is not to wear any jewelry that dangles or makes noise. Perfumed lotions or colognes should not be used because they tend to cause nausea in people who are ill. Patients have a "clean and crisp" image of nurses, and they judge the nurse's competence by looks and behavior.

---

**Giving a Report**

BOX **2.9**

Organize your thoughts using an outline format before giving your report to the staff nurse assigned to your patient. Provide the following information briefly and professionally:

- Patient name and room number
- Condition of patient (any changes), last vital signs, oxygen saturation
- Diagnostic tests or surgery undergone or both
- Treatments or procedures performed (including bath)
- As-needed (PRN) medications given and effect
- Intake and output (I&O) if ordered
- If intravenous (IV) administration bag will need changing
- Appearance of IV sites and locations
- Tubes in place and whether functioning properly; output
- Appearance of wounds and dressings in place; wound drainage output
- Bowel sounds: present or absent?
- Whether patient has had a bowel movement
- Voiding status
- Any abnormalities of heart or lung sounds
- Pain or comfort status
- Any patient concerns
- Use the SBAR format as appropriate: **S**–situation, **B**–background, **A**–assessment, **R**–recommendation

## SMOKING

If a nursing student smokes during a break, a breath freshener should be used before returning to the bedside; the smell of cigarettes is offensive to an ill nonsmoker. Cigarette smell is also carried on clothes back into patient areas. It is unprofessional to subject an ill person to this odor. Many facilities are completely smoke free and have no areas where smoking is permitted. It might be a good time to quit the habit. Ask about resources available for smoking cessation in your student health center.

## DRESS

Student nurses are expected to dress professionally whenever they enter the clinical facility. This includes if students need to go to the units to obtain the data needed for their patient assignments. Although uniforms are not usually required when you are going to the hospital to gather patient data, a clean, pressed laboratory coat worn over professional clothes and a name tag are required. Jeans, shorts, mini-skirts, T-shirts with slogans, sandals, spiked high-heeled shoes, cowboy boots, and other such casual attire are inappropriate.

It is not considered professional to wear a nursing uniform when out with friends for a drink or shopping after the day's work is done. People do not know whether you have just finished a shift or are about to go on duty. A uniform worn while working in a clinical setting can be contaminated with many types of bacteria. It is best to change before running errands on the way home. The uniform should be worn only to and from the clinical area or work and while you are on duty. A freshly laundered uniform is to be worn each clinical day.

## Behavior

Behavior can add to your professional image or detract from it. Your facial expression, body language, and posture are components of your overall image. Chewing gum or eating while providing patient care is considered unprofessional. A cheerful smile, modulated voice, erect posture, and body language that indicate attentive listening and quiet efficiency instill a feeling of confidence in patients.

### PREPARATION

Professional behavior also includes being well prepared for the clinical experience and turning in completed written work when it is due. Instructors expect students to come to the clinical experience on time, in correct attire, and with the tools of the trade—a working watch, a stethoscope, a pen, and a name tag and badge.

### ENVIRONMENTAL NEATNESS

Attention to environmental care of the assigned patients' units and to the nurses' stations and workrooms is another facet of professional behavior. Patient areas should be straightened at least once a shift. When time permits, add water to flowers to keep them fresh. Clean up after yourself in the medication room and at the nurses' station. Wipe up spills, throw away trash, and put equipment back where it belongs.

### ATTENDANCE AND PUNCTUALITY

Most nursing instructors consider the clinical experience equivalent to reporting to work. Absence is excused only for illness or a family emergency. It is not professional to miss your clinical day to study for an examination or to take care of outside business matters. However, students are expected to remain at home if they are ill with a condition that is contagious, such as a cold with fever, constant sneezing, coughing, or runny nose. Intestinal influenza symptoms of vomiting or diarrhea should also signal the student to stay home. Exposing patients or colleagues to additional illness is not professional. Know how to notify your instructor that you will not be in attendance. Most schools or boards of nursing require a set number of clinical hours to be completed. Missed clinical time will most likely need to be made up.

### COST CONTAINMENT

Think cost effectively. Check the patient's room for needed dressing or procedure supplies before taking new items from the clean supply area, to ensure that the least amount of supplies are used. Continually ask yourself whether there is a less expensive way to do the procedure. Do not take unneeded linen into the patient's room: anything not used still has to be laundered. Remember to charge out supplies you use for the patient as required.

## Verbalization

Appropriate verbalization is the third component of the professional image. Stress is usually high for the nursing student when in the clinical setting. It is necessary to make a conscious effort to stop and think before speaking when under such stress. Try to develop some quick stress relief techniques that you can use to calm yourself in particularly stressful situations (see Chapter 3). When you are with patients or staff, it is better to say too little than too much. Be aware of any nervous habits you might have, such as talking too much or too loudly or giggling, and curtail the behavior when it starts.

## PATIENT PRIVACY

Remembering to provide privacy when interviewing a patient or performing a procedure builds trust between the patient and the nurse. Keeping your voice low when in the halls or at the nurses' station helps maintain the restful atmosphere that patients need. Try to provide maximum privacy in semi-private rooms when interviewing a patient. When giving medications, be sure to identify visitors in the patient room and get permission from the patient to continue with medication administration. Giving medications includes explaining the medications and their purpose, which may disclose the patient's diagnosis or other protected information.

## COURTESY

Be courteous to other health care workers, as well as to patients. Saying, "May I," "Please," and "Thank you," and refraining from directly interrupting another contribute to a professional image. Call the patient Mr., Mrs., or Ms. unless given permission to use his or her first name. Do not use "honey," "dear," or other such terms. Consideration of others is essential to professional behavior. You are there to meet the patient's needs, not to socialize. Keeping conversation and attention focused on the patient rather than on you or outside activities is best. Students should not gather together during clinical hours. Time is to be spent with the patients, studying their charts, or interacting with other health care professionals for the purpose of collaboration or learning.

## NONJUDGMENTAL ATTITUDE

Another aspect of professionalism is development of a nonjudgmental attitude toward patients and staff. Students sometimes find fault with nurses who do things differently from how their nursing school is teaching them. There are many right ways to perform different tasks. If the principles of asepsis and safety are followed, there is nothing wrong with performing a procedure in a different sequence or in a different way. Before loudly proclaiming that a nurse is doing something wrong, it is wise to discuss the matter quietly with the instructor.

## CULTURAL SENSITIVITY

Patients and staff are not to be judged according to the student's values or cultural beliefs. Through the clinical learning process, students will become familiar with and learn to respect the values and beliefs of other cultures and individuals. To care for patients of different cultures, you must learn about the practices of cultural groups other than your own. By inquiring about cultural practices you observe, you can learn a great deal. There are many articles on usual practices within a variety of cultural groups. Several practical handbooks are also available. Assessment of cultural preferences should be part of your nursing care. Never assume that just because a patient is part of a particular ethnic group, he or she adheres to that group's cultural practices. You must assess rather than assume. Culture extends beyond ethnicity into families and social groups. The role of the nurse is to deliver professional, competent care to patients, taking into consideration the patient's personal values and practices while not allowing bias to alter care delivery. The nurse should be able to care for patients whose family relationships, sexual orientation, and religious beliefs are different from his or her own.

## REPORTING PROBLEMS

If something has occurred with a patient that violates the principles of asepsis or safety, pointing it out to the instructor is the professional response. Current peer review criteria require that questionable practices or incidents be brought to the attention of the nurse involved and the supervisor. However, when you are in the student role, allowing the instructor to handle such matters is best.

## HONESTY

Honesty is essential to professionalism. Students are encouraged to admit mistakes and be honest with everything that they do, including their written work. It is unprofessional to compose someone else's nursing care plans or other written assignments or to have others contribute to yours. There are times when good students are encouraged to assist those having trouble with written work. Discuss the guidelines for this type of activity with the instructor before giving or getting assistance.

Professional behavior includes resisting passing along information on test questions to students in other class sections or allowing other students to copy from your answers. Such behavior is considered as much a form of cheating as copying answers from another student's examination.

Incorporating professionalism into your behavior and nursing practice occurs over time. You will benefit from observing the image, behavior, and verbalization of nurses whom you perceive as being highly professional and then attempting to model yourself accordingly.

## ■ CLINICAL EVALUATION

Each nursing school has a form used to evaluate student performance in the clinical setting. Become familiar with this form during the first week of the semester. In addition, find the list of clinical objectives for the semester and review them each week to be sure you are meeting them.

### Basic Competence

Initially, students are evaluated on their mastery of basic competence for particular skills. There often is a formal check-off evaluation period for various required skills in the skills laboratory before the student ever attempts the skill in the clinical setting. Usually a skill is either passed or failed. If the student does not pass the skill check-off evaluation, remediation and practice are necessary before a second chance is given to pass the skill.

Once the student is caring for patients in a clinical setting, informal evaluation takes place on a weekly basis. This means that students are evaluated for competence and consistency of correct performance of skills previously evaluated in the skills laboratory or for adherence to principles taught in the lecture class. (Some schools do not have a skills laboratory.) General concepts that are always undergoing constant evaluation, once they have been covered in theory class, include the use of medical asepsis, communication, safety, legalities of practice, organization, and time management.

As content regarding various body systems is covered in theory class, the instructor will be evaluating your ability to apply the principles you have learned in the clinical setting. For example, once you have covered the basic concepts of disease and nursing care for the urinary system, you will be expected to be able to assist a patient to urinate, check for a full bladder, realize when a patient has gone too long without emptying the bladder, recognize signs that might indicate an infection, and determine when the color of urine is abnormal. **Students sometimes fail to understand that they are going to be evaluated on synthesis and application of knowledge as well as on the performance of skills.**

If you have difficulty in the clinical area and very often find that things do not seem to be going right, immediately ask your instructor to meet with you to find out specifically what you can do to redirect the course of events. Admitting mistakes, taking positive steps to correct deficiencies, and being honest will cause your instructor to evaluate you on your progress rather than on individual situations during which things went wrong. In other words, you will be seen in a favorable light when you exhibit these behaviors.

Instructors often verbally tell students how they are doing every few weeks; if you do not get this type of feedback, ask for it. Try asking, "How am I doing? Is there any area in which you see that I need to improve to be at a passing level?" This feedback will help you relax more and stop worrying about what the instructor may be thinking.

## Clinical Written Work

The evaluation of clinical written work is based on instructor expectations and course requirements. Items on the evaluation form usually indicate what will be evaluated on written work. For example, "Writes individualized problem statements/nursing diagnoses pertinent to each patient's condition and problems" may be one item on the evaluation form. This requirement is appropriate for a first-semester student. Progress toward meeting this requirement is shown by writing one or two correct problem statements or nursing diagnoses on the first nursing care plan, writing two or three correct problems on the next care plan, and writing correct problem statements/nursing diagnoses covering all of the patient's basic needs for the final care plan of the semester.

By the final course, the evaluation form might state, "Writes comprehensive problem statements/nursing diagnoses in order of priority for assigned patients, considering psychosocial aspects of care as well as physical condition and problems."

It is helpful to ask your instructor for a sample of the type and level of written work desired. This sample provides you with an image of what is expected. Each nursing instructor has particular ideas about how the various parts of the nursing care plan should be written. Some instructors place more emphasis on one part than on another. It is to your benefit to find out specifically what each instructor wants before you turn in your first assignment.

If there is a grading form to be used for the written work you are going to turn in, consult it to see that you have included everything that is required before completing the assignment. You do not want to lose points simply because you forgot to complete a section of the assignment.

## Formal Evaluation

A formal, summary type of evaluation is usually performed at set intervals during the semester. At these times, the instructor will fill out the evaluation form and set a conference time to review it with you. Often you will be asked to perform a similar self-evaluation. Asking at the beginning of the semester whether a learning period and a specific evaluation period will be offered is best; you will then know what to expect. At formal evaluation time, you will be evaluated on your achievement of the objectives for the clinical experience as well as for each item on the evaluation form. Usually a minimum level of competency is expected from students at each level. This level is often defined by the course objectives. Instructors look for progress toward the course objectives as well as for consistency in adherence to the principles taught. If you do not feel that you understand the evaluation form, ask for a conference with your instructor during the first 2 weeks of school to clarify what is required of you.

# DEALING WITH STRESS

3

## ■ CONTROLLING STRESS LEVELS

Becoming a nursing student automatically increases stress levels because of the complexity of the information to be learned and applied and because of new constraints on time. There are several ways you can consciously decrease the stress associated with school. One way is to become very organized so that assignment deadlines or tests do not come as sudden surprises. By following a consistent plan for studying and completing assignments, you can stay on top of requirements and thereby prevent added stress. Carry as few units as possible to lighten the study load.

### Set Priorities

Another way to decrease stress while in school is to set personal priorities. Take time to survey all outside obligations and determine what can be given up during nursing school. Perhaps it would be best to concentrate solely on school if you are single and on school and family if you are married or a parent. That may mean restricting your social life or giving up many social activities such as being a scout leader, Sunday school teacher, room mother at school, chief carpool driver, soccer coach, or Little League organizer. When school is completed, these extra roles can be taken up again. Adopt the motto "Keep It Simple" for your life while in school. The fewer outside distractions and responsibilities you have, the better your chances for success. Do not let housemates or dorm mates constantly distract you.

### Ask for Help

If you have home responsibilities, consider asking for assistance from family and friends during your school years. A lot of stress can be reduced if someone else will take over carpool duties for school-age children. Relatives and good friends may be willing to help with this task. A spouse may be able to help if work schedules permit. Relatives can act as representatives once in a while at a child's school function that falls on the evening before an important test. All household members can help with housekeeping, cooking, and errands. Adolescents can grocery shop from a list, and children from the age of 9 years can prepare a simple dinner, even if it is hot dogs, scrambled eggs and biscuits, or frozen dinners cooked in the microwave oven. Children can prepare their own school lunches and can fix yours, too! Things do not have to be perfect for these few years of school. Let go of ideals regarding meals and the state of living quarters or yard. The goal is to keep all occupants healthy and in touch with one another while you get through school. When a relative or dear friend asks what you would like for a special occasion gift, tell him or her that you would like a maid service to clean the house really well or a gardener to do some yard work or to take care of some other major chore. Be creative with gift requests; ask for what you really need to decrease your stress.

## Tackle One Task at a Time

Try to decrease your workload and maximize your time by handling items only once. Most of us spend a lot of time picking up things we put down rather than putting them away when we have them in hand. Going straight to the closet with your coat when you come in instead of throwing it on a chair saves you the time of hanging it up later. Discarding junk mail immediately and filing the rest of your bills and mail as they come in rather than creating an ever-growing stack saves time when you need to find something quickly. Filing all items requiring further attention in some fashion helps you remember to take care of things on time rather than being so engrossed in your schoolwork that you forget about them. Many nursing students have had their power or telephone service cut off because the bill simply was forgotten or buried in a pile of old mail.

## Exercise

Regular exercise, even if only a 10-minute brisk walk each day, aids in reducing stress. Although you may have been able to enjoy regular sessions at the health club or at an exercise class several times a week, you now may have to cut down on that time without giving up a set schedule for an exercise routine. Using an exercise bicycle that has a book rack on it at home, the YMCA, or a health club can help you accomplish two goals at once: You can exercise while beginning a reading assignment or while studying notes for an exam. Listening to lecture recordings while doing floor exercises is another option. At least a couple of times a week, however, the exercise routine should be done without the mental connection to school; time for the mind to unwind is necessary, too.

## Stop for 10 Minutes

Taking 10 minutes a day for yourself is very beneficial for stress reduction. Closing yourself in your room, lying down with eyes shut, and just free floating for a few minutes can revive energy and stop the whirlwind of thoughts of family obligations or nonstop tasks that tend to increase stress. Reading a few pages of a magazine or a book, listening to favorite music, napping for a short time, or doing a relaxation technique between the time you reach home and begin the evening routine can refresh both the body and the mind.

## Focus on Now

Another technique to help keep stress levels at a minimum is to stop worrying about things that cannot be changed. A great deal of energy is spent by many people on worrying about a situation that has not yet taken place. There will be time enough to worry about an event once it has actually occurred. Check yourself and ask whether you are a person who spends precious energy in this fashion. Wouldn't you rather spend that energy elsewhere? All of your "preworry" most likely will not change the event. Worrying about whether your teenager will have an accident while driving will not prevent such an event or cause it to happen. Worrying about whether a completed assignment will be graded favorably will not affect the grade; what is done is done. Try to focus on this day and this time, and do not worry about problems ahead of time. Deal with problems as they occur; if you cross a bridge before you need to, you will be paying the toll twice.

## Change Your Perception

Donald Tubesing, in his book *Kicking Your Stress Habits* (1992), talks about using the technique of relabeling (reframing) to alter stress from bad to good. (This book is still in print.) The author explains that the effect of an experience on you is determined by how you label it. You have a choice as to how you view things. Labeling your clinical experience as exciting and challenging will make it far less stressful than labeling it as frightening and forbidding. If you label events as adverse during your daily crises, you end up with a batch of problems by the end of the day; if you label the same events as challenges, you end up with a bunch of opportunities. When something really seems stressful, ask yourself, "Will this matter in another 12 months? In 5 years?" This technique can quickly place things in a broader perspective.

### Practice Self-Affirmation

A helpful method for decreasing test stress is to practice self-affirmation. After you have adequately studied and really know the material, stop and look in the mirror each time you pass one and say to yourself—preferably out loud—"I know this material, and I will do well on the test." After several times of watching and hearing yourself reaffirm your knowledge, you will gain inner confidence and be able to perform much better during the test period. This technique really works for students who are adventurous enough to use it. It may feel silly at first, but if it works, who cares? It will work for performing skills in clinical as well, as long as you have practiced the skill sufficiently.

### Become More Assertive

Learn to stand up for your rights without violating the rights of others. Do not let people "walk all over you," because that leads to frustration, anger, and stress. Assertive techniques take practice, but a school counselor can help you get started. You will learn to show understanding of the other person's feelings but be able to assertively state what you need. Assertiveness is essential to becoming a patient advocate. (See Chapter 6 for Internet resources on assertiveness.)

### Find Humor

Laughter is a great stress reliever. Watching a short program that makes you laugh, reading something funny, or sharing humor with friends helps decrease stress. Sometimes just putting a humorous twist on something that you are finding stressful relieves the stressed feeling. If you can manage to laugh many times a day, your stress levels should fall.

### Refuel and Recharge

The old standbys of enough sleep and adequate nutritional intake also help keep excessive stress at bay. Although nursing students learn about the body's energy needs in anatomy and physiology classes, somehow they tend to forget that glucose is necessary for brain cells to work. Skipping breakfast or lunch or surviving on junk food puts the brain at a disadvantage. How can you expect to grasp material while reading textbooks if your brain is operating in a glucose-deficient mode? Can you perform in a top-notch manner in the clinical setting if the last meal was more than 8 hours ago? A car is not expected to run without gas; why should a body, and especially a brain, be expected to perform correctly when there is no fuel on board?

Once nursing classes start you will probably not be able to obtain the same amount of sleep as you did before, but rest is essential to the body and brain for good performance. Think of it as recharging the battery. A run-down battery provides only substandard performance. For most students, it is better to spend

7 hours sleeping and 3 hours studying than to cut sleep to 6 hours and study 4 hours. The improvement in the rested mind's efficiency will balance out the difference in the time spent studying. Knowing your natural body rhythms is necessary when it comes to determining the amount of sleep needed for personal learning efficiency.

## Know Your Internal Clock

Determine whether you are a "lark" or an "owl." Larks—day people—do best getting up early and studying during daylight hours. Owls—night people—are more alert after dark and can remain up late at night studying, catching up on needed sleep during daylight hours. It is better to work with natural biorhythms than to try to conform to an arbitrary schedule. You will absorb material more quickly and retain it better if you use your most alert periods of each day for study. Of course, it is necessary to work around class and clinical schedules. Owls should attempt to register in afternoon or evening classes and clinical sections; larks do better with morning classes and day clinical sections.

## Other Stress Remedies

- Take a walk.
- Play with a pet.
- Sit quietly and contemplate nature.
- Get a shoulder, back, or foot massage.
- Take a hot bath or shower.
- Talk out a stressful situation with a close friend.
- Write your thoughts and feelings in a journal.

# ■ STRESSES UNIQUE TO NURSING

## Danger of Infection

Becoming a nursing student brings special situations that many find very stressful. Nurses care for patients with chronic or terminal diseases. Many diseases patients have can be contracted by the nurse. Also, patients do not always get well; sometimes they lose body functions or die, an event that causes students considerable grief. The following paragraphs present some information and suggestions for decreasing the fear of contracting harmful diseases and for dealing with dying patients.

### PREVENTING CONTRACTION OF DISEASE

All health facilities use Standard Precautions to prevent health care workers from contracting harmful organisms through patient contact or spreading infectious material between patients. The goal of Standard Precautions is to establish a barrier between the patient and anything that may transmit organisms to the worker or others. Personal protective equipment (PPE) such as gloves, masks, gowns, and goggles are used when exposure to pathogenic organisms or body fluids that may contain them is possible. Because it is not known which patients may harbor these harmful agents, all patients are considered to be potential carriers, and Standard Precautions are used for every patient. Gloves are used while working with patients when there is any chance of coming into contact with blood, other body fluids, and secretions. Dressings and linens may be contaminated, and you should wear gloves when handling these items. Box 3.1 presents a synopsis of the Centers for Disease Control and Prevention's Standard Precautions.

## Standard Precautions

BOX **3.1**

The Centers for Disease Control and Prevention (CDC) recommends using Standard Precautions, formerly known as Standard Blood and Body Fluid Precautions, for the care of all patients. These precautions are directed at preventing parenteral, mucous membrane, and nonintact skin exposures of health care workers to blood-borne pathogens such as human immunodeficiency virus (HIV), hepatitis B virus (HBV), and hepatitis C virus (HCV). Current medication therapy can delay or eliminate the onset of acquired immunodeficiency syndrome (AIDS) from HIV, but there is no cure or vaccination at this time. Because HBV and HCV cause serious illness (chronic hepatitis) and are known to predispose the patient to cancer of the liver, immunization with HBV vaccine is recommended as an important adjunct to Standard Precautions for health care workers who may be exposed to blood. There is no vaccine for hepatitis C. Other infection control measures are used in addition to Standard Precautions. The following is a summary of the CDC guidelines.

### BODY FLUIDS

Use Standard Precautions for all body fluids and tissues. Blood is the single most important source of HIV, HBV, HCV, and other blood-borne pathogens in the health care facility. Standard Precautions are used in the presence of feces, nasal secretions, sputum, tears, urine, and vomitus. General infection control measures apply to the handling of these body fluids. Proper hand hygiene is mandatory.

### GENERAL PRECAUTIONS

1. Use Standard Precautions for all patients.
2. Routinely use appropriate barrier precautions when contact with blood or other body fluids of any patient is anticipated.
   - Do not reuse gloves.
   - Do not wash or disinfect surgical or examination gloves for reuse.
3. Take precautions to prevent injuries caused by needles, scalpels, and other sharp instruments or devices during procedures; when cleaning used instruments; when disposing of used needles; and when handling sharp instruments after procedures.
   - Discard needles uncapped and unbroken after use.
   - Place disposable syringes and needles, scalpel blades, and other sharp items in puncture-resistant containers.
   - Place puncture-resistant containers as close as practical to the areas in which sharp items are used.
4. Barrier devices should be used for mouth-to-mouth resuscitation, or a resuscitation bag should be used.

### HAND HYGIENE

Hand hygiene is the hallmark of preventing the spread of infectious organisms. The CDC has recently modified the hand hygiene guidelines.

- Wash the hands with an antimicrobial soap and water any time they are visibly soiled. Wash hands with antimicrobial soap and water if contact with spores (e.g., *Clostridium difficile* or *Bacillus anthracis*) is likely to have occurred. Alcohols, chlorhexidine, iodophors, and other antiseptic agents have poor activity against spores.
- An approved alcohol-based hand rub is recommended for hand hygiene when hands are not visibly soiled:
  - immediately after removing gloves.
  - between patient contacts and when otherwise indicated to avoid transferring microorganisms to other patients or environments.

## Standard Precautions (cont'd)

- between tasks and procedures on one body area before moving to another body area on the same patient to prevent cross-contamination of different body sites.
- before entering and when leaving a patient room.
▪ Do not wear artificial fingernails or extenders when providing direct patient contact.

### USE OF PERSONAL PROTECTIVE EQUIPMENT
▪ Use appropriate barrier methods—gloves, surgical mask, protective eyewear, face shield, gown, and apron—when participating in invasive procedures.
▪ Wear appropriate personal protective equipment (PPE) when the nature of the patient contact indicates that contact with blood or body fluids may occur.
▪ Wear gloves when touching blood and body fluids, mucous membranes, or nonintact skin, or when handling items or surfaces soiled with blood or body fluids. When performing skin sticks such as injections, finger or heel sticks, venipuncture, and other vascular access procedures, use nonpermeable gloves.
▪ Change gloves after contact with each patient, and perform hand hygiene.
▪ Change gloves during patient care if the hands will move from a contaminated body site (e.g., perineal or wound area) to a clean body site.
▪ Wear impermeable gowns or aprons during procedures that are likely to generate splashes of blood or other body fluids.
▪ Wear masks and protective eyewear or face shields during procedures that are likely to generate drops of blood or other body fluids to prevent exposure of mucous membranes of the mouth, nose, and eyes.
▪ Wear a gown for direct patient contact if the patient has uncontained secretions or excretions; do not reuse gowns.
▪ Prevent contamination of clothing and skin during the process of removing PPE.
▪ When performing or assisting in a delivery, wear gloves and a gown when handling the placenta or the infant until blood and amniotic fluid have been removed from the infant's skin, and use gloves during postdelivery care of the umbilical cord.
▪ If a needle stick occurs through a glove or a glove becomes torn, remove it and wash with soap and water. Notify your supervisor.

### TRANSMISSION-BASED PRECAUTIONS
▪ Contact Precautions—used when the infectious organism is transmitted by direct contact. Gloves and gowns are used when in direct contact with the patient or the patient's environment.
▪ Droplet Precautions—used when the infectious organism is transmitted via droplets usually expelled from the respiratory system by coughing or sneezing. Masks are worn when in close contact with the patient. If significant spray of respiratory fluids is anticipated, wear gowns and full facial protection.
▪ Airborne Precautions—used when the infectious organism remains suspended in the air for long periods. A special airborne infection isolation room is needed. Any health care personnel entering the room must use a previously fit-tested N95 respirator mask or alternate positive airflow hood. Use gloves for touching contaminated items. If spraying of respiratory secretions is possible, gowns should be worn.

### RESPIRATORY HYGIENE AND COUGH ETIQUETTE
▪ Cover the mouth and nose when sneezing or coughing, preferably coughing or sneezing into the crook of the elbow rather than into the hands.
▪ Use a mask when in patient care areas if a respiratory problem is causing a runny nose, coughing, or sneezing.
▪ Perform hand hygiene when hands have been in contact with respiratory secretions or have used tissues.

Continued

Dealing with Stress

## Standard Precautions (cont'd)

### ENVIRONMENTAL CONSIDERATIONS

- Standard sterilization and disinfection procedures currently recommended for use in health care settings are adequate.
- Sterilize instruments or devices that enter sterile tissue or the vascular system before reuse.
- Clean and remove soiled areas on walls, floors, and other surfaces routinely; extraordinary attempts to disinfect or sterilize are not necessary.
- Use chemical germicides approved as hospital disinfectants and tuberculocides to decontaminate spills of blood and other body fluids. In the absence of a commercial germicide, a solution of sodium hypochlorite (i.e., household bleach) in a 1:10 dilution is effective.

### PRECAUTIONS WITH SOILED LINENS

- Handle soiled linen as little as possible and with minimum agitation to prevent gross microbial contamination of the air and of persons handling the linen.
- Place linen soiled with blood or body fluids in leak-resistant biohazard bags at the location at which it was used.

### HANDLING SPECIMENS

- Place all specimens of blood and listed body fluids in well-constructed containers with secure lids to prevent leakage during transport; place specimens in a marked biohazard bag.
- Be careful not to contaminate the outside of the container when collecting specimens.

### INFECTIVE WASTE DISPOSAL

- Incinerate or autoclave infective waste before disposal in a sanitary landfill.
- Dispose of containers of secretions as biohazardous waste in specially marked bags or containers.

Adapted from Siegel JD, Rhinehart E, Jackson M, et al: *Guideline for isolation precautions: preventing transmission of infectious agents in healthcare settings 2007*, Atlanta, 2007, Centers for Disease Control and Prevention, Healthcare Infection Control Practices Advisory Committee.

## BASIC SELF-PROTECTION

Self-protection against all disease is provided by following all infection control guidelines within the clinical facility. Recognize that the nursing profession by its very nature will cause you to come in contact with communicable diseases. New organisms and diseases are continually emerging. *Good hand hygiene* is the most effective method of reducing transfer of microorganisms from one person or object to another. Following Standard Precautions by washing hands or using hand sanitizer after each patient contact, before gloving, and when you remove gloves is one way to help decrease exposure to harmful organisms.

It is preferable to use nitrile rather than latex gloves because many people develop an allergy to latex.

Several drug-resistant microorganisms are encountered in the hospital and the community. Methicillin-resistant *Staphylococcus aureus* (MRSA) and vancomycin-resistant enterococci (VRE), as well as the *Clostridium difficile* organism, can cause very serious infections. Follow CDC recommendations and facility protocols for isolation precautions based on the mode of transmission. Strictly adhering to Standard Precautions at work and practicing good asepsis at home and in the community setting will protect you.

Keeping the immune system in top functioning order should be another priority for every nursing student and nurse. This is accomplished by getting sufficient sleep, eating properly balanced meals, exercising regularly, attending to minor illnesses quickly, and keeping stress levels within limits. Along with the use of Standard Precautions, boosting the immune system is the best protection against communicable diseases.

## Working with Patients Who Are Dying

First experiences with patients who are dying are very stressful for most students. Prepare yourself by knowing what you can do to help the patient. Be familiar with the stages of grief and dying, while realizing that each patient deals with impending death individually. The nurse's role is to provide basic care for and comfort to the patient. Attend to small tasks such as lubricating lips, straightening linen, offering a back rub or a foot rub, straightening the environment, making certain enough warmth is provided, and offering sips of fluid, for example. Provide adequate pain relief and provide comfort measures. Check with the patient about what he or she desires.

Psychologically, assist the patient through the stages of the coping process; help the patient face issues as honestly as possible by being supportive. All you need to do in this area is to let the patient know that you are available to talk about whatever is pertinent. Never force a subject on the patient. Be honest and ask questions cautiously about what the patient knows and feels. Take cues from the patient about what topics are acceptable to explore. Do not avoid the issues of the illness, complications, or impending death. The patient may need to talk to someone not personally involved.

Sometimes it is helpful to reminisce with the patient, going through his or her life and remembering the major landmarks and fun times. Encourage family members or significant others to remember the past with the patient as well. Best of all, just offer yourself by simply being there for the patient. Check his or her needs often, and offer to just sit quietly in the room as time permits.

If the patient is not fully awake or aware, many of these nursing actions can be helpful to the family. Watching a loved one go through the dying process is difficult, and the presence and support of the nurse can help ease some of the distress the family may be experiencing.

Discuss any fears you have with your instructor. Be specific about questioning what to do in certain situations. Know what to expect with a particular patient as death approaches. Will breathing become labored? Will the skin become mottled? Will the patient become unconscious? Ask the nurse who is caring for the patient about the probable course for this patient. Knowing what to expect can greatly decrease your fear of the actual event. Also clarify your role in the event that the patient stops breathing or has a cardiac arrest. Usually you should stay with the patient and use the call system to call out for the primary nurse or charge nurse. Always determine whether the patient has a do-not-resuscitate (DNR) order. **If such an order has not been written, you must begin cardiopulmonary resuscitation as soon as a respiratory or cardiac arrest is observed, even though it is known that the patient is terminally ill.**

## High-Acuity-Level Patients

The pace in acute care settings is fast, and patients in the hospital are much sicker than 20 years ago. The acuity level is often quite high, and patients have multiple problems, lines, tubes, and equipment in use as well as numerous medications to be administered. The best way to decrease the stress when assigned such patients, or multiple patients, is to stay focused on each patient and to be well prepared. Learn to anticipate possible patient events, such as deteriorating condition, infiltrated IV site, and complications common to the disorder.

## Special Patient Situations

Being prepared to deal with patients who are depressed, hostile, aggressive, or manipulative can also help decrease stress on clinical days. Your nursing texts tell you how to determine whether a patient is depressed or manipulative, but you will probably be able to pick out hostile and aggressive patient behaviors through your own life experiences.

### DEPRESSED PATIENTS
Nursing interventions that sometimes help depressed patients include the following:

- Quietly sit with the patient.
- Encourage performance of activities of daily living; assist as needed.
- Work slowly; be patient and gentle.
- Point out the patient's strengths and accomplishments; emphasize good qualities.
- Do not admonish the patient to "cheer up and look at the bright side of things"; do not be overly bright and cheerful.
- Encourage social interaction, particularly exercise.
- Be alert for signs of self-destruction and the potential for suicide.

All patients seen in the emergency department or admitted to the hospital must be screened for suicide risk. The Joint Commission has issued guidelines for identifying those at risk and interventions to help. See https://www.jointcommission.org/assets/1/18/SEA_56_Suicide.pdf for full details.

Report findings indicating risk to your charge nurse and instructor.

### MANIPULATIVE PATIENTS
Manipulative patients use a variety of means to get what they want from the nurse. This behavior has various causes. It may be the way the patient has learned to communicate or respond to stress; often the patient simply fears losing control. Some specific nursing interventions useful in dealing with the manipulative patient include the following:

- Respond to the inappropriate behavior as calmly as possible; set limits. If the patient is shouting, explain that shouting is inappropriate, is disturbing to other patients, and makes it impossible to help. Say, "Please stop shouting, and tell me how I can help you."
- Be consistent and firm. State how often you can check on him or her; restate this information as needed when a demand is made between scheduled times.
- Do not become defensive; do your best not to take insults personally. Establish a personal emotional distance but not a professional distance.
- Be aware of how this behavior affects you. The patient may remind you of previous experiences with manipulative family members or friends.
- When all else fails or if you get into a loud exchange indicating demanding behavior, tell the patient you are leaving the room because of his or her behavior and that you will be back when he or she has calmed down. State when you will be back, and then arrive on time.

## HOSTILE PATIENTS

Hostile, aggressive behavior includes verbal or physical threats. This type of behavior is usually an attempt to maintain control over the situation. When another person becomes aggressive, the usual response is to become defensive. At times, aggressive behavior occurs in family members as well as in patients. Some helpful nursing interventions to use when these behaviors occur include the following:

- Let the person know you are aware of his or her anger; allow feelings to be expressed freely. Ask what is upsetting the person and inquire what can be done to help him or her feel less angry and frustrated. Actively listen. Do not place blame.
- Provide the opportunity for the patient to make suggestions about self-care; give in to demands that are not unreasonable.
- Encourage as much physical activity as possible to help release pent-up feelings.
- Allow the patient to make decisions and choices regarding his or her care or the timing of procedures and tasks of daily living. This provides a sense of power and control.
- Rather than responding to the content of what the person is ranting about, attempt to respond to the underlying feelings.
- When a patient raises his or her voice, lower yours. Treat the person as an adult.
- Do not make promises that cannot be kept. This destroys trust.

Protect your safety if a situation escalates by taking the following actions:

- Maintain a safe distance from the patient while verbally interacting (at least an arm and a half's length away); maintain eye contact.
- Position yourself between the patient and the exit; keep your hands in sight.
- Remove potential weapons from the patient's reach; remove any item from around your neck.
- Know how to summon help.

## THE PATIENT WHO HAS DIFFICULTY COMMUNICATING VERBALLY

You may find it stressful to be assigned to care for a patient who is aphasic and has difficulty communicating as a result of disease or brain injury from a stroke or head trauma. There are several different varieties of aphasia (e.g., expressive, receptive, global, mixed), and patients can experience the problem from a slight to a profound degree. Your nursing texts can give you specific suggestions for dealing with individual types of aphasia, but here are some general guidelines:

- Keep the environment as relaxed and quiet as possible.
- Assume that the patient can understand what is heard even though his or her speech is jargon (nonsensical) or the patient is mute.
- Speak to the patient on an adult level; do not treat the patient as mentally incompetent.
- Talk to the patient, not about the patient to someone else in the room.
- Face the patient, establish eye contact, and speak slowly and distinctly without dropping your voice level at the end of sentences. Do not shout.
- Give short, simple directions; use pantomime and body language to enhance the words.

- Phrase questions so that they can be answered with a yes or no, and look for nonverbal behavior that agrees with the patient's answer.
- Give the person time to respond to questions; processing may be slower than usual.
- Do not ask more than one question at a time.
- If there is a need to repeat something, use the same words the second time. If difficulty still exists, phrase what was said differently.
- Allow only one person to speak at a time.
- Be very patient.

Remember that the person may get very frustrated when unable to verbalize adequately. A statement such as, "It must be very difficult and frustrating not to be able to make people understand what you want to say" and a caring touch may help. An understanding of what it must be like for the person may help keep you from becoming short and impatient. Be aware that aphasia worsens with anxiety or fatigue.

## Personal Safety

Nurses often work shift hours and must travel in the dark. General safety rules for driving and walking, such as these, should be followed:

- Keep car doors locked at all times.
- Have the car door key or release out and ready before you depart from the building.
- Look in the back seat before entering the car.
- Be certain to keep the gas tank at least one quarter full at all times. Keep the car in good running condition.
- Travel on well-lighted, busy streets, avoiding isolated back roads and troubled parts of town.
- If you are being followed, drive to the nearest open business for help or drive to a police or fire station.
- Park only in areas that are well lighted. When leaving the clinical facility, walk with several other people or ask the security guard to accompany you during early morning or nighttime hours.
- Do not stop to aid a stranger in a stalled vehicle; proceed to an open business and report the stalled vehicle to the police.
- If you have vehicle trouble, raise the hood, get back into your vehicle, and lock it. Turn on the flashers. When someone offers assistance, roll down the window only enough to talk. Never get into a stranger's car.
- Avoid walking alone. When you walk, do not keep looking down; walk with your head up and shoulders back, and survey your surroundings; make eye contact with passersby.
- Stay in well-lighted, pedestrian-traveled areas. Avoid shortcuts through alleys, parks, vacant lots, and deserted areas.
- If someone stops and asks for directions, maintain your distance; especially, do not approach a stopped car.
- If you are being followed, briskly walk to the nearest business or residence for help.
- If you are bothered by people in a car, turn and walk the other way.
- Women should hold a purse close and securely; avoid carrying extra money and valuables.

- Have your door key ready before leaving your car to enter your home.
- Be alert; note the people around you, your surroundings, and the total environment. Texting or talking on a cell phone distracts you from being aware of your surroundings.

## SEXUAL ASSAULT PREVENTION AND RESPONSE

Classes in personal defense are offered at most colleges and in many communities. A few hours spent learning methods of self-defense can prevent injury or rape. Following the preceding safety tips when walking and driving also can help prevent sexual assault. However, should you be threatened with rape or assault, there are some things that may prevent its occurrence. Active resistance is one way, and it must be used quickly. The purpose is to startle or surprise your attacker. For active resistance, use whatever you have as a weapon. Kick, use your elbow, scream, yell, or run; use your keys, purse, or whatever you have. A spray device with mace, tear gas, or pepper is effective, and nurses or students who have to walk to distant parking lots would be wise to have such a device in hand before leaving the building. Most such devices attach to a key ring.

Should rape occur, call the police immediately. In addition, call the local rape crisis center for quick counseling and a support person. It is important not to take a bath or shower. Physical evidence, including seminal fluid, hairs, scrapings of flesh from under fingernails, and any of the attacker's blood on the victim, is necessary for positive identification of the attacker and a court conviction. The police will ask for information about the car the attacker was driving, including make, color, and license plate number; the attacker's race, approximate age, weight, height, color and length of hair, and color of eyes; clothing the attacker was wearing, including hat, tie, shirt, pants, shoes, and glasses; and any unusual marks, scars, tattoos, piercings, or rings. Knowing whether the attacker is right handed or left handed is also helpful. Although statistically women are more likely to be victims of sexual assault than men, it can happen to anyone.

## ■ SELF-ASSESSMENT

### Assessing Your Stress Level

Sometimes, no matter what stress reduction techniques are used, the stresses of keeping up with classes, clinical, family, and job can become too much. Keep a finger on the pulse of your stress by assessing your stress status about once a month. Ask the following questions:

- Are you easily angered by uncontrollable events such as being put on hold on the telephone, traffic jams, persistent poor weather patterns, or malfunctioning equipment?
- Do you feel rushed all the time because tasks seem to never end?
- Has your sleep pattern changed? Do you have difficulty falling or staying asleep?
- Has your eating pattern changed? Have you lost or gained weight?
- Are you tired, anxious, or feeling "burned out" all the time?
- Do you suffer from chronic headaches, backaches, stiff neck or shoulder, or intestinal or stomach complaints?
- Do you often find yourself clenching or grinding your teeth?
- Are you drinking or smoking more than usual?

- Do you often lose your temper or burst into tears without a good reason?
- Are you constantly irritable?

## Addressing Your Stress

If the answer is "yes" to three or more of the preceding questions, sit down and evaluate how you can decrease the stress levels in your life. If you do not believe you can change anything, seek professional assistance. Counseling is available at your school, from instructors, school counselors, and the school health center. You pay for these services when you register for your classes, so use them. Do not wait to go for help. The quicker you resolve the problem, the better your chance for success in school.

Using a relaxation technique will help you keep stress levels under control (Boxes 3.2 and 3.3). However, to be useful, the technique must be used regularly several times a week until using it becomes second nature.

---

### Guided Imagery for Relaxation

BOX **3.2**

This is a sample script for a guided imagery experience. It can be recorded and replayed while doing the exercise. Writing your own script and recording it maximizes the experience. When recording your script, read slowly in a soft but audible voice. Pause sufficiently after each instruction and section to allow time for following the instruction or forming the mental image. Performing this guided imagery exercise regularly can reduce stress.

When performing the exercise, sit or lie down and stretch out. Reduce noise and other distractions as much as possible. Dimming the light in the room is beneficial.

**SCRIPT**

- Close your eyes and gently relax.
- Take a deep, slow breath. Feel your lungs fill with clean, fresh air. Slowly exhale, sending all tension out with the air you exhale.
- Take another deep, slow breath; let it out slowly, sending body tension with it.
- Visualize yourself walking on a path in the woods at the edge of a meadow.
- Smell the clean air, the forest, and the flowers in the meadow.
- Feel the warmth of the sun and the soft, warm breeze. Hear the crunch of pine needles under your feet. It is so peaceful and serene here.
- You approach a brook, gently gurgling over the rocks in its path. You listen to the pleasant sound of the running water. It is almost as if the brook talks to you, welcoming you to this beautiful place of peace, comfort, and serenity.
- You look at the grass and moss growing in beautiful greens beneath the water.
- Patches of sunlight filtering through the trees warm your body. What a perfect spot to enjoy.
- You find a comfortable place, spread the blanket you were carrying, and sit and gaze at the trees, the meadow, and the blue sky with fluffy white clouds slowly moving to the horizon. What a beautiful place.
- You listen to the birds calling to each other and contemplate their cheerful melodies.
- A butterfly flits across your field of vision. You watch it as it zigzags across the meadow, going from flower to flower.
- It is so warm, pleasant, and peaceful here. You remember other days in similar surroundings.
- You concentrate on the feelings of warmth and peace the sun and breeze convey to you. Happiness fills your heart and soul, and you realize you can return here anytime you wish. This place is yours.

## Guided Imagery for Relaxation (cont'd)

- Replenished, you arise, fold the blanket, and prepare to return up the path.
- You look around you once more—at the trees, the meadow, the sky, and the brook—imprinting the scene in your memory to take with you. This is your special place; it will always be here for you.
- You walk slowly up the path through the sunlight toward home.
- When you are ready, open your eyes.

## Relaxation Exercise

BOX **3.3**

This exercise is performed by recording the following script and following the instructions as it is played. Using the exercise regularly over a period of weeks makes it easier to call on these techniques to induce relaxation during an exam or at other times you feel particularly tense.

Slowly read the script in a soft, firm voice. Allow sufficient pauses between segments for the instructions to be followed. Sit in a chair or lie down to do the exercise. Decrease outside noise and distractions as much as possible.

**SCRIPT**

- Close your eyes and find something to focus on mentally. It may be a spot of light, your pulse, a visual image, or whatever you choose. Try to hold it constant.
- Breathe in slowly and deeply; hold it a moment, and slowly breathe out. Now breathe normally, slowly, in and out.
- Tighten the muscles in your face and neck as firmly as you can, while clenching your teeth. Feel the tension. Hold it; slowly relax the muscles. Feel the relaxation in your face, jaw, and neck.
- With less tension, tighten the muscles in the face, jaw, and neck again. Feel this level of tension. Let go and relax. Notice the feeling of relaxation.
- Tighten the muscles in your chest firmly. Hold it; feel the tension. Let the chest muscles relax. Notice the difference between the tension and relaxation.
- With less tension, tighten the chest muscles again. Now let the muscles relax. Feel the relaxation.
- Tighten the fists and arm muscles as hard as possible. Hold the tension a moment. Slowly relax the muscles. Notice the difference in feeling between tension and relaxation.
- With less tension, tighten the fists and arm muscles again. Hold it. Let the muscles relax. Feel the relaxation.
- Tighten the abdominal muscles firmly. Hold the tension, noting the feeling. Relax the muscles, noting the difference between tension and relaxation.
- With less tension, tighten the abdominal muscles again. Hold it. Allow the muscles to relax completely. Notice the feeling of relaxation.
- Tighten the muscles in your right leg and foot. Hold the tension. Note the feeling. Allow the muscles to relax. Notice the difference between tension and relaxation.
- With less tension, tighten the muscles in your right leg and foot again. Hold it. Completely let go of the tension in the muscles and relax. Feel the relaxation.
- Tighten the muscles in your left leg and foot firmly. Hold it. Note the tension. Allow the muscles to relax. Focus on the difference between tension and relaxation.
- With less tension, tighten the muscles in your left leg and foot again. Hold it. Completely let go of the tension in the muscles and relax. Notice the feeling of relaxation.
- Breathe in and out deeply and slowly five times, focusing on your breathing.
- When you are ready, open your eyes.

# CONTINUING YOUR EDUCATION

# 4

## ■ TAKING THE NEXT STEP

### Types of Programs

Some colleges offer a ladder program within the nursing division. Some programs begin with a certified nursing assistant (CNA) curriculum that progresses to a 1-year practical nurse program. When this 1-year program is completed, the student has the option to complete a second year for an Associate Degree in Nursing (ADN) or continue for a Bachelor of Science in Nursing (BSN) degree.

A number of colleges and universities offer a BSN completion program for ADN graduates. In these programs it generally takes 1 to 1½ years to complete the nursing part of the curriculum. The completion program can be accomplished via online and distance learning. Today many colleges and universities offer online learning, condensed programs, and many other options for varied student needs.

Traditional BSN programs require 4 to 5 years to complete. These programs usually provide a more rounded education with required courses in the arts and sciences. The nursing courses usually do not begin until after the first 2 years of study. Students who are already licensed nurses may receive credit for some previous nursing courses. A Master of Science in Nursing (MSN) and a Doctor of Nursing Practice (DNP) degree can also be obtained by online and distance learning in many instances once a BSN has been earned. Some schools offer a BSN by online learning to graduates with degrees in other health-related fields.

The following four ways are available to evaluate an RN-to-BSN program or a BSN/MSN-to-DNP program:

1. Check the amount of general education units required. You should not have to repeat courses you have already successfully completed.
2. Look at the number of nursing courses required. Again, you should not have to repeat coursework you have already completed in a previous program.
3. Check the courses required and the amount of time required to earn the degree.
4. Calculate the entire cost of the program. Consider the cost of textbooks and any required travel.

### Returning Students

Returning to school is a big step. If you have been in the workforce for many years, the student role will be a bigger adjustment for you than for those who recently graduated from a nursing program. The written work required for ADN, BSN, or BSN completion programs is extensive, and a heavy emphasis is placed on the nursing process, concept-based learning, and evidence-based practice. You will review the nursing process during the first few weeks of class. Do your best to develop a good understanding of each component, how it works, and how the five parts are integrated with the application of the whole circular process. Spending time now to review the nursing process, especially as it relates to paperwork, will save you considerable time and frustration in your nursing classes and clinical courses. Explore how to research evidence-based nursing care.

## Differences in Training

An even greater emphasis will be placed on the development and use of critical thinking throughout your nursing courses. If you graduated many years ago and have been working as a licensed nurse, studying critical thinking skills would be wise. Most fundamentals of nursing texts address this content. Several good books aimed particularly at critical thinking in nursing are available on the market. An example is *Critical Thinking and Clinical Judgment: A Practical Approach to Outcome-Focused Thinking*, 6th edition (2017), by Rosalinda Alfaro-LeFevre.

The RN student is expected to learn in-depth assessment skills. Emphasis will be placed on extensive history taking and skillful, thorough physical assessment. Compared with the licensed practical nurse/licensed vocational nurse (LPN/LVN), the RN is expected to develop even greater expertise in identifying problems and detecting complications and changes in a patient's condition. If it has been some time since you have used all your physical assessment techniques, practicing them on friends and relatives is the best way to brush up and improve your skills.

The BSN student studies more in-depth supervisory and management content than the ADN student. The BSN student is also trained in community health and research techniques. A course in statistics is usually required. Some BSN curricula require more science and mathematics courses as well.

## Differences in Curriculum and Demands

Your ADN or BSN curriculum is similar to the previous nursing curriculum but more comprehensive. The volume of reading is time consuming, and much written work must be completed. Try to cut your work schedule to 20 hours a week or less. Aim for success from the beginning. If you have spare time and see that your class average is good after working part time for a while, you can slowly increase your work hours. Only rarely can students with family commitments be successful in an RN program while working full time. Many single students who do not have other obligations have difficulty keeping up with school if they try to work 40 hours per week. Students who are single parents often need to work more hours, but they are at a disadvantage because they are the only caregivers for their families, which seriously limits available study time. Relatives can sometimes be asked to take total charge of the children for several hours, thereby providing blocks of study time one or more times a week for the months you are in school.

## Bringing Skills and Habits with You

Depending on where you have been working, you will have some advantages over new nursing students. If you have been working in a hospital or long-term care facility, you should be confident and competent with skills such as administering medications, catheterization, and nasogastric tube insertion. You should also have an advantage in that you are familiar with many prescription drugs.

Sometimes instructors prefer that a skill be performed differently from how you learned it years earlier. Protocols and ideas on the best way to do things change from time to time as new information emerges on evidence-based nursing practice. If you learned a procedure differently in your previous nursing courses, you may have to practice outside of class to learn to perform the skill in a new way.

Continuing Your Education

If you have been working in home care and regularly using your assessment skills, you may have an advantage over other students in this area. You can function independently and make decisions, and you have developed good people skills and know how to adapt to various situations.

If you have been working in a long-term care facility, you are very familiar with the problems and needs of older adults and with the ways of efficiently caring for this population. For example, you know the techniques that are helpful in administering medications to the person who has a decreased ability to swallow, how to distract the patient who has decided not to do what you want him or her to do, and how to quickly clean up the bed and skin of a patient who is incontinent.

If you have years of experience in a surgical department, you are comfortable and confident with sterile techniques. You have an idea why the patient has postoperative pain and why joints and muscles are sore and stiff after a lengthy operation. You are familiar with the routine of assisting with a cardiac or respiratory arrest.

## Catching up with Generic Students

Unless you work in an area in which you manage a variety of drugs, you will need to spend extra time refreshing your pharmacological knowledge when you enter an ADN or a BSN program. Generic students may have had many months to study drugs. You should start refreshing your memory about a set number of drugs each week from the first week. Learn the drugs first by classification and then by family group. If you understand how the class of drugs works, you can determine the possible side effects and then determine the probable nursing implications. After you have learned the classification information, choose individual drugs that differ in side effects or nursing implications from the general drugs of the class, and learn those.

One problem many returning students have is adopting the role of a student when they are in a clinical setting. Each student should clarify with the instructor which skills can be performed without supervision and which skills the instructor must be called on to observe. Although performing a procedure while working as a licensed nurse is so natural, as a student, you might easily forget that you cannot simply just do it. Get into the "think before doing" mode during your clinical experience hours.

## Role Transformation

As you near the end of the RN curriculum, you will be learning more advanced supervision of others. Advanced leadership skills are part of the RN competencies. Sometimes a practical nurse who has little supervisory experience may find it difficult to act in a leadership role. One way to prepare for leadership is to observe continually how the charge nurse and staff RNs interact and delegate tasks to the other personnel on the unit. Role-play for yourself how you would handle various situations and assignments within your daily work routine. Observe the nuances of supervision in action.

The BSN student should begin to see the larger picture from the standpoint of administration and the institution. This perspective requires a broadened mind-set. For an ADN, the focus is on providing patient care. For a BSN, the focus expands to include the needs of the nursing unit and the institution as well as the patient. Aspects of the new role include learning to schedule personnel, managing conflicts among staff, writing policies, and performing evaluations of staff. A greater emphasis is put on long-term quality improvement.

Try to mainstream yourself with all the students rather than segregating yourself with other returning practical nurses or ADNs. In this way you can glean information that other students learned during their courses for which you received credit because of your previous nursing classes. You can find out which instructors may suit your needs and personality the best, and you will have some assistance in refining your paperwork from those who have already been through some of the assignments. Share your expertise when asked; it will boost your morale. You have a lot to offer to the learning experience of the group.

Success begins with planning. Consistently using a planner (such as this one) for scheduling your time for study, exams, classes, and other activities can help you achieve success in the nursing program, whether you are a returning practical nurse, an ADN, or a beginning BSN student.

Continuing Your
Education

# CLINICAL QUICK REFERENCE

# 5

## ■ COMMUNICATION

### Prefixes and Suffixes Used in Medical Terms

| Term | Meaning | Term | Meaning |
|------|---------|------|---------|
| **Combining Forms** | | myo- | muscle |
| adeno- | gland | naso- | nose |
| alveolo- | air sac | nephro- | kidney |
| andro- | man, male | neuro- | nerve |
| angio- | vessel | onco- | mass, tumor |
| appendic/o- | appendix | oophoro- | ovary |
| arthro- | joint | ophthalmo- | eye |
| audio- | hearing | orchio- | testis |
| bio- | life | osteo- | bone |
| broncho- | bronchus | oto- | ear |
| carcino- | cancerous | patho- | disease |
| cardio- | heart | pharyngo- | pharynx |
| ceco- | cecum | pneumo- | lung, air |
| cephalo- | head | procto- | rectum, anus |
| cerebro- | brain | prostato- | prostate |
| cervico- | neck | psycho- | mind |
| chole- | bile | pyelo- | kidney |
| cholecysto- | gallbladder | radi- | ray, radiation |
| claviculo- | clavicle | rhino- | nose |
| colo- | colon | salpingo- | tube |
| cranio- | skull | spleno- | spleen |
| cutaneo- | skin | stoma- | mouth |
| cysto- | bladder, sac | thrombo- | clot |
| dermato- | skin | thyro- | thyroid |
| duodeno- | duodenum | tracheo- | trachea |
| encephalo- | brain | tricho- | hair |
| entero- | intestine | uretero- | ureter |
| erythro- | red | uro- | urine |
| esophago- | esophagus | vertebro- | vertebra |
| gastro- | stomach | | |
| gingivo- | gums | **Prefixes** | |
| gluco- | sugar | a-, an- | without, away from, not, no |
| gyneco- | woman | | |
| hemato- | blood | ab- | away from, absent |
| hepato- | liver | ana- | up, back, again |
| hystero- | uterus | ante- | before |
| laryngo- | larynx | auto- | self |
| leuko- | white | bi- | two, twice |
| lipo- | fat | co-, con- | with, together |
| meningo- | membrane | contra- | opposite, against |
| myelo- | marrow, spinal cord | dia- | through, complete |

## Prefixes and Suffixes Used in Medical Terms—cont'd

| Term | Meaning | Term | Meaning |
|------|---------|------|---------|
| dys- | difficult, painful, abnormal | -ia | condition |
| | | -iasis | morbid condition |
| ec-, ecto- | outside, out | -ic | pertaining to |
| endo-, ento- | within | -ist | one who specializes in |
| epi- | above | -itis | inflammation |
| exo- | out | -logy | process of study |
| hyper- | excessive, above | -lysis | dissolution, setting free |
| hypo- | below, deficient | | |
| meta- | change, over, after | -malacia | softening, soft |
| peri- | around, surrounding, about | -megaly | enlargement |
| | | -oid | form, shape |
| pro- | before, in front of | -ology | study or science of |
| re- | back, again | -oma | tumor |
| retro- | behind, backward | -opsy | viewing |
| sym-, syn- | together, with | -osis | condition, disease |
| trans- | across, through, beyond | -pathy | disease, suffering |
| | | -penia | deficiency, lack of, decrease |
| **Suffixes** | | -pexy | fixation |
| -ac | pertaining to | -plasty | mold, shape, repair |
| -al | pertaining to | -ptosis | downward displacement, falling |
| -algia | painful condition, pain | | |
| -cele | hernia, swelling, sac | -rhea | flow, discharge |
| -centesis | puncture of a cavity | -scope | instrument to visually examine |
| -cyte | cell | | |
| -desis | fusion, binding, fixation | -scopy | process of examining |
| | | -sis | state of, condition |
| -ectasis | expansion, dilation | -spasm | involuntary spasm |
| -ectomy | excision, removal of a body part | -stasis | control, constant level |
| | | -stomy | creation of an opening |
| -emia | blood | -therapy | treatment |
| -genic | origin, formation | -tome | instrument for cutting |
| -gram | the record made, mark | -tomy | process of cutting |
| -graph | instrument for recording, machine | -trophy | nourishment |
| -graphy | the process, process of recording | | |

Adapted from O'Toole M, editor: *Dictionary of medicine, nursing, and health professions*, ed 10, St Louis, 2017, Mosby.

## SBAR Communication Tool

The intent of the *SBAR* tool is to overcome communication barriers between doctors and nurses, between nurses, and between nurses and other health care professionals. It can help prevent care lapses and mistakes when the patient is handed off from one nurse to another or when the patient is transferred to another unit or facility. The acronym provides a quick and concise method of conveying detailed information in incident or emergency situations. The acronym stands for **S**ituation, **B**ackground, **A**ssessment, **R**ecommendation or **R**equest. Here is an example:

Clinical Quick Reference

S:    Dr. Savoy, this is Nurse Lopez at ABC Extended Care Facility.
Mr. Tanglewood is an 85-year-old with Alzheimer's disease. He tripped
in the bathroom and bumped his head on the toilet about 30 minutes
ago. One of the nursing assistants saw him trip; there was no loss of
consciousness at any time.

B:    He is normally alert and oriented to person, and he routinely ambulates.

A:    His blood pressure is 140/83, pulse 75, respirations 16 per min. He has
a 3-cm laceration and hematoma just superior to his left eyebrow. The
bleeding was readily controlled with direct pressure. We have applied
an ice pack and pressure bandage over the wound. He is alert, and his
speech is clear and appropriate to his baseline. He denies any pain, and
he does not seem to have tenderness or bruising except on his forehead,
but he did extend his right hand to break his fall.

R:    Could I get an order to have him transported to the emergency
department for additional evaluation and treatment? And do you have
any additional orders for Mr. Tanglewood?

Adapted from Williams P: *Fundamental concepts and skills for nursing*, ed 5, St Louis, 2018, Saunders.

## Basic Phrases in English and Spanish

| Question or Phrase in English | Question or Phrase in Spanish | Phonetic Pronunciation |
|---|---|---|
| Do you speak English? | ¿Habla usted inglés? | AH-blah oo-STEHD een-GLEHS? |
| I don't understand. | No entiendo. | noh ehn-t-YEHN-doh. |
| My name is … | Me llamo … | meh YAH-moh … |
| What is your name? | ¿Cuál es su nombre? | kwahl ez soo NOM-bray? |
| Speak more slowly, please. | Hable más despacio, por favor. | AH-bleh mahs deh-spah-SEE-yoh, pohr fah-VOHR. |
| I'm here to help you. | Estoy aquí para ayudarle. | ehs-TOY ah-KEE PAH-rah ah-yoo-DAHR-leh. |
| I'm going to take your vital signs. | Le voy a tomar los signos vitales. | leh voy ah toh-MAHR lohs SEEG-nohs vee-TAH-lehs. |
| I'm going to take your pulse. | Le voy a tomar el pulso. | leh voy ah toh-MAHR ehl POOL-soh. |
| I'm going to take your blood pressure. | Le voy a tomar la presión. | leh voy ah toh-MAHR lah preh-SYOHN. |
| I'm going to take your temperature. | Le voy a tomar su temperatura. | leh voy ah toh-MAHR soo tehm-peh-rah-TOO-rah. |
| Do you understand? | ¿Entiende usted? | ehn-t-YEHN-deh oo-STEHD? |
| Are you allergic to anything? | ¿Es usted alérgico(a) a cualquier cosa? | ehs oo-STEHD ah-LEHR-hee-koh(kah) ah kwahl-kee-YEHR KOH-sah? |
| Do you take any medications? | ¿Toma medicamentos? | TOH-mah meh-dee-kah-MEHN-tohs? |
| Here is the call light. | Aquí está la luz para llamar a la enfermera. | ah-KEE eh-STAH lah looss PAH-rah yah-MAHR ah lah ehn-fehr-MEH-rah. |
| This is the television control. | Este es el control de la televisión. | EHS-teh ehs ehl kohn-TROHL deh lah teh-leh-vee-see-YOHN. |
| This is the bed control. | Este es el control de la cama. | EHS-teh ehs ehl kohn-TROHL deh lah KAH-mah. |

## Basic Phrases in English and Spanish—cont'd

| Question or Phrase in English | Question or Phrase in Spanish | Phonetic Pronunciation |
|---|---|---|
| Don't get out of bed by yourself. | No se baje de la cama solo(a). | noh seh BAH-heh deh lah KAH-mah SOH-loh(ah). |
| You may not eat or drink anything more before surgery. | No comerá o beberá nada antes de la cirujía. | Noh koh-meh-RAH oh beh-beh-RAH NAH-dah AHN-tehs deh lah see-roo-HEE-ah. |
| Do you have pain? | ¿Tiene dolor? | t-YEH-neh doh-LOHR? |
| Are you nauseated? | ¿Siente el estómago revuelto? | s-EHN-teh ehl ehs-TOH-mah-goh reh-VWEHL-toh? |
| Take a deep breath in, please. Exhale. | Respire profundo, por favor. Exhale. | reh-SPEE-reh proh-FOON-doh, pohr fah-VOHR. ehks-AH-leh. |
| Now cough. | Ahora tosa. | ah-OR-a TOH-sah. |
| I am going to give you an injection. | Le voy a poner una inyección. | leh voy ah poh-NEHR OO-nah een-yehk-see-YOHN. |
| I have some medications for you to take. | Tengo unas medicamentos para que usted las tome. | TEHN-goh OO-nahs meh-dee-kah-MEHN-tohs PAH-rah keh oo-STEHD lahs TOH-meh. |
| When was your last bowel movement? | ¿Cuándo tuvo último excremento? | KWAHN-doh TOO-voh soo OOL-tee-moh ehks-kreh-MEHN-toh? |
| I need to measure your urine. | Debo medir su orina. | DAY-bow meh-DEER soo oh-REE-nah. |
| It is time for your bath. | Es hora de su baño. | ehs OH-rah deh soo BAHN-yoh. |
| Do not pull on the tube. | No jale el tubo. | noh HAH-leh el TOO-boh. |
| Sit up, please. | Siéntese, por favor. | s-YEHN-teh-seh, pohr fav-VOHR. |

Clinical Quick Reference

# ■ BASIC PRINCIPLES OF NURSING CARE

## The Nursing Process

The five-step nursing process (pictured on the inside front cover) is set in motion at the time of the initial assessment. There is continuous interaction among the components, and the patient is the focus of all activities within the process. Arrows point in both directions, indicating that the process is always in motion. Thus each component is subject to revision as new information is obtained through interaction with the patient. Following are some examples of activities used within each step of the nursing process.

## ASSESSMENT
- Data gathering
  - Initial admission assessment
  - Interview and history taking
  - Physical examination/assessment
  - Measure vital signs
  - Chart review

- Beginning of shift, quick head-to-toe assessment
- Focused assessment for major problem (e.g., respiratory, cardiac, neurologic)
- Assessment of equipment needed for a procedure
- Assessment of learning needs
- Review of literature
- Review of anatomy and physiology of body systems involved in patient problem
- Read about disease process or surgery
- Consult other health team members for further information

## NURSING DIAGNOSIS
- Analysis of data to determine problem areas
- Definition of problems
- Formulation of problem statements/nursing diagnoses (RN)
- Recognition of appropriate problem statements/nursing diagnoses chosen for care plan (LPN/LVN)
- Collaboration with patient for prioritization of problems/nursing diagnoses

## PLANNING
- Write goals/expected outcomes for each problem.
- Set a time for expected outcomes to be met.
- Plan interventions to assist patient to meet expected outcomes or achieve goals.
- Devise a teaching plan.
- Check physician's orders to see what has to be done.
- Plan ahead for surgical care.
- Plan ahead for medication administration.
  - Check to see that medications are on the unit.
  - Verify medication orders on the medication administration record (MAR) with the physician's original orders.
- Collaborate with other health team members to plan patient's total care for the shift.
- Document the nursing care plan.
- Plan revision of interventions when evaluation indicates the need.
- Plan work organization for the shift.

## IMPLEMENTATION
- Supervise implementation of the nursing care plan.
- Carry out planned nursing interventions.
- Delegate/assign tasks to ancillary nursing personnel.
- Perform skills and procedures.
  - Measure and record intake and output (I&O).
  - Change a dressing.
  - Check equipment in use.
  - Apply a heat treatment.
  - Give medications.
- Teach patients.
- Counsel assigned patients and families.
- Consult/collaborate with other health team members (e.g., social worker, dietitian, pharmacist, physician).

## EVALUATION

- Evaluate patient condition.
- Evaluate effect of nursing interventions.
- Determine whether nursing interventions are helping patient meet expected outcomes/goals.
- Evaluate data to see whether there is progress toward recovery.
- Evaluate whether interventions have to be revised.
- Evaluate effect of treatments.
- Evaluate for side effects and therapeutic effect of medications.
- Document evaluation data.
- Evaluate whether work organization schedule has to be revised.

## Documentation

### DESCRIPTIVE TERMS USED IN DOCUMENTATION

| Word | Idea to Be Charted | Terms Suggested |
|---|---|---|
| Abdomen | Appearance | Distended, round, flat, soft, firm, hard, rigid, protruding, flaccid, tympanic, tender, boardlike, bruised, or ecchymotic |
| Bleeding | In very large amounts or spurts | Spurting blood, profuse oozing |
| | Very little | Minimal amount; scant |
| | Location | Blood in vomitus (hematemesis), blood in urine (hematuria), blood in sputum, nosebleed (epistaxis), or black tarry stool (melena) |
| Breath | Taking air in | Inspiration |
| | Breathing air out | Expiration, exhalation |
| | Short time without breathing | Apnea |
| | Rapid breathing | Hyperpnea |
| | Cannot breathe lying down | Orthopnea |
| | Snoring sounds of breathing | Stertorous respiration |
| | Unpleasant odor | Halitosis |
| | Increasing dyspnea with periods of nonbreathing | Cheyne-Stokes respirations |
| | Difficulty breathing or labored breathing | Dyspnea, respiratory distress |
| Cough | Various types of coughing | Tight, loose, deep, dry, hacking, painful, exhaustive, hollow |
| | Coughs all the time | Continuous |
| | Coughs over long period of time | Persistent |
| | Coughs up material | Productive |
| | Coughs without producing material | Nonproductive |
| | Sudden attacks of coughing | Paroxysmal |
| Consciousness | Aware of surroundings | Alert—conversant, fully awake, and conscious |
| | Partly conscious | Groggy, lethargic, semiconscious |
| | Arousable but not conscious; responds to some stimuli | Stuporous, semiconscious; responsive to verbal stimuli, responsive to tactile stimuli |
| | Unconscious, cannot be aroused; does not respond to stimuli | Comatose |

Continued

Clinical Quick Reference

## DESCRIPTIVE TERMS USED IN DOCUMENTATION—cont'd

| Word | Idea to Be Charted | Terms Suggested |
|------|--------------------|-----------------|
| Convulsion | Muscles contract and relax | Clonic tremor or convulsion |
| | Muscle contraction maintained for a time | Tonic tremor or convulsion |
| | Localized muscle contraction | Spasm, twitch |
| | Begins without warning | Sudden onset |
| | Abrupt start and end of spasm or convulsive seizure | Paroxysm |
| Drainage | Water from the nose | Coryza |
| | Sticky | Viscous |
| | Bloody | Sanguineous |
| | Contains serum and blood | Serosanguineous |
| | Fecal (contains bowel material) | Fecal |
| | Contains mucus and pus | Mucopurulent |
| | From vagina after delivery | Lochia |
| Odor | Not pleasant; pungent | Aromatic |
| | Spicy like fruit | Fruity |
| | Unpleasant | Offensive; foul |
| | Smelling like a particular thing | Characteristic of … |
| Pain | Amount of pain | Use statement of patient; slight to severe; rate on a scale of 1 to 10 |
| | Types of pain | Aching, dull, slight, burning, throbbing, gnawing, acute, chronic, generalized, superficial, excruciating, unyielding, cramping, darting, colicky, continuous, shifting, agonizing, piercing, intense, cutting, transient, localized, remittent, persistent |
| | Comes in seizures | Spasmodic |
| | Spreads to certain areas | Radiating |
| | Begins suddenly | Sudden onset |
| | Hurts when moving | Increased by movement |
| Skin | Terms to describe condition | Pale, pink, red, moist, dry, clear, coarse, tanned, scaly, thick, loose, rough, tight, infected, discolored, jaundiced, mottled, calloused, edematous, excoriated, abraded, bruised, painful, scarred, black, oily, yellow, brown, white, clammy, rash, wrinkled, smooth |
| Speech | Unable to be understood | Incoherent |
| | Meaningless | Rambling, irrelevant |
| | Runs words together | Slurs |
| | Difficulty in speaking | Dysphasia |
| | Unable to speak | Aphasia |
| | Other terms to describe | Stammering, stuttering, hoarse, feeble, fluent, clear |

## HIPAA Considerations for Nurses

To follow the privacy rules outlined in the Health Insurance Portability and Accountability Act (HIPAA) and protect patients' privacy:

- Avoid discussion with patients about their condition within earshot of other patients or visitors. Use a low voice or take the patient to a private area for verbal interaction.
- Remove the patient record from the computer screen when you leave. Be certain that other patients or visitors cannot see the screen while you are working.
- Use only patients' initials on worksheets, assignment sheets, and student care plans and assignments.
- Do not discuss patients in the elevators, cafeteria, or other public locations, even with your same-unit personnel.
- Do not discuss patients with your family and friends at any time.
- Do not divulge patient information to patient's family or others without explicit patient permission.
- HIPAA privacy requirements state that patient information concerning name, age, diagnosis, and other personal information should not be posted. Paper charts and medication records must be kept in a confidential area.

## Discharge

### PATIENT TEACHING

Cover the following points when performing discharge teaching:

- Care of incision, if present
- Dressing changes, supplies, techniques, soiled dressing disposal
- Care of tubes, drain suction devices, other equipment in place
- Care of intravenous (IV) site, role of the patient and family, role of the home health nurse
- Activity level permitted; restrictions
- When patient can return to work
- Driving restrictions
- Sexual activity guidelines
- Weight-lifting restrictions
- Bathing/showering precautions
- Rest requirements
- Diet guidelines; any restrictions
- Signs and symptoms to report
- When and where to make a follow-up appointment
- Medications, purpose, schedule, side effects to report
- Where to obtain medical equipment to be rented or purchased
- Number to call if questions arise

### WRITING A DISCHARGE SUMMARY

Follow your agency's format and guidelines regarding content. The following points are usually included in the discharge summary, which is written in the nurse's notes or on a discharge sheet or electronic health record (EHR) flow sheet:

- Who received the teaching (patient, patient and family, family caregiver, etc.)
- A summary of the patient's care

- An outline of all patient teaching, including what the patient was taught about diagnosis, diet, activity, medications, wound care, special care, signs and symptoms of complications to report to the physician, use of medical equipment, follow-up care, and referrals
- Documentation that the patient understands the teaching and that written instructions have been given to him or her
- Any exceptional details or unusual findings regarding the illness or present condition
- Condition of the patient at the time of discharge
- Description of status of wounds, dressings, drains, and tubes still in place
- Where patient is told to call and the phone numbers should further help be needed

## Standard Reference Materials

These references may be in book form on the units but are often online in the system computers or can be obtained by a mobile device app:

**Drug reference:** Contains information on drugs organized by generic name, brand name, or category of use. Use it to find pertinent information about drugs you will be giving.

**Procedures manual/skills manual:** Contains the accepted procedures for performing various nursing skills in the clinical facility. This thick book is an in-house volume and may vary in content from one clinical facility to another. Use it to review each nursing procedure (e.g., urinary catheterization, sterile dressing change) before preparing to perform the procedure.

**Diet manual:** Lists the foods allowed and forbidden on the various therapeutic diets available in the clinical facility. Use this manual to check what the patient may and may not have when a special diet is prescribed.

**Documentation/charting manual:** Designates the accepted procedures and forms to be used for documenting nursing care within the particular clinical facility. Use this manual to learn to correctly document the nursing care you give.

**Medical dictionary:** Provides definitions of medical terms, pronunciation of words, correct spelling of medical words, lists of abbreviations, and a variety of appendices that may include lists of symbols, prefixes and suffixes, nursing diagnoses, diagnosis-related groups (DRGs), tables of laboratory values, foreign language terms, anatomic tables or charts, food value charts, and other helpful aids.

## General Steps for All Procedures

For all procedures, the following elements should be performed before the procedure is started:

- Check the physician's order.
- Obtain a signed consent form if required.
- Carry out any patient preparation necessary prior to the procedure.
- Gather equipment.
- Verify the patient's identity using two identifiers (name, birth date).
- Obtain assistance if necessary (e.g., someone to hold patient).
- Provide privacy (e.g., close door, drape as appropriate).
- Explain the procedure to the patient.
- Obtain consent to proceed (verbal or implied for routine nursing procedures).

- Arrange work space as needed.
- Perform hand hygiene.

For all procedures, the following should be performed at the end of the procedure:

- Assess response to procedure (e.g., "Does the catheter hurt?").
- Ensure safety; bed in low position (side rails up if needed).
- Rearrange environment for patient's convenience and comfort (call bell within reach).
- Thank patient and give any special instructions related to procedure.
- Dispose of equipment.
- Perform hand hygiene.
- Document procedure and patient response.

### Guidelines for Cast Care

- Check the cast for integrity: no breaks, cracks, crumbling edges.
- Assess the degree of tightness around the casted part: it should not be cutting into the flesh.
- **Assess for circulation and movement distal to the cast: check pulses, skin temperature, ability to move joints, and sensation.**
- Assess for any pain related to the placement of the cast.
- Feel along the cast for "hot" spots that might indicate underlying infection.
- Smell the ends of the cast for any odor, which may indicate the presence of infection.
- Position the casted area per the physician's orders; support joints proximal and distal to the cast.
- Supervise range-of-motion exercises for joints proximal or distal to the cast as ordered.
- Caution patient not to poke anything under the cast.
- Handle a cast that is still wet with the flat of the palm of the hand rather than the fingertips when positioning.
- Listen to what the patient says and respond to any complaints with further exploration of the problem.

## ■ ASSESSMENT QUICK REFERENCE

### Blood Pressure Parameters and Classifications

| Classification | Systolic Measurement (mm Hg) | | Diastolic Measurement (mm Hg) |
|---|---|---|---|
| Normal | <120 | and | <80 |
| Prehypertension | 120-139 | or | 80-89 |
| Stage I hypertension | 140-159 | or | 90-99 |
| Stage II hypertension | ≥160 | or | ≥100 |

### Neurologic Assessment

All patients should be routinely assessed for level of consciousness, orientation, and thought processes. Clinical facilities, especially long-term or psychiatric settings, are likely to have expanded versions of the mental status examination.

## ORIENTATION AND MENTAL STATUS

### Orientation

- What place is this?
- What is the date?
- What city do you live in?
- What is your husband/wife's name?

### Ability to follow simple instructions

- Hold out your left hand with the palm up.
- Please hand me the _____ (pen, pencil, book; providing free choice of several objects; also tests object recognition).

### Memory

- Do you remember my name? (If so, what is it?)
- What did you have for breakfast this morning?

**Delirium and dementia.** Use the mnemonic *JAMCO* to assess for delirium or dementia:

- **J**udgment—Does the patient have insight into own behavior? Is the patient aware of danger or safety issues?
- **A**ffect—Is affect blunt, flat, inappropriate, suddenly changed, or variable?
- **M**emory—Is memory intact? Does the patient have remote memory, but not recent or immediate? Is memory better during the day?
- **C**ognition—Is the patient able to process abstract thoughts? Are thoughts fragmented or disorganized? Does the patient make up answers to questions (confabulate) to hide deficits?
- **O**rientation—Is the patient oriented to person, place, and time? Does the patient recognize family and friends?

## GLASGOW COMA SCALE

The Glasgow Coma Scale is used to assess the condition of patients who have a decreased level of consciousness or who are at risk for a decreasing level of consciousness or neurologic injury. Assess each category of response, and add up the score.

| Category of Response | Stimulus | Response | Score* |
|---|---|---|---|
| Eye opening | Approach to bedside | Spontaneous response | 4 |
| | Verbal command | Opening of eyes to name or command | 3 |
| | Pain | Opening of eyes only to pain | 2 |
| | | Lack of eye opening to any stimulus | 1 |
| Best verbal response | Verbal questioning with maximum arousal | Appropriate orientation; conversant; correct identification of self, year, month, and place | 5 |
| | | Confusion, disorientation in one or more areas, but is conversant | 4 |
| | | Inappropriate use of words, cursing, lack of sustained conversation | 3 |
| | | Incomprehensible words, moaning | 2 |
| | | Lack of sound with any stimuli | 1 |

## GLASGOW COMA SCALE—cont'd

| Category of Response | Stimulus | Response | Score* |
|---|---|---|---|
| Best motor response | Verbal command[†] | Obedience to the command | 6 |
| | Pain (pressure on proximal nail bed) | Lack of obedience but attempts to remove offending stimulus | 5 |
| | | Flexion withdrawal | 4 |
| | | Abnormal flexion, flexing of arm at elbow and pronation, making a fist | 3 |
| | | Abnormal extension, extension of arm at elbow with adduction and internal rotation of arm at shoulder | 2 |
| | | Lack of response | 1 |

*The highest possible score is 15. The higher the score, the better the condition of the patient.

†For example, "Raise your arm, hold up two fingers."

Adapted from Lewis SM, Bucher L, Heitkemper MM, et al: *Medical-surgical nursing: assessment and management of clinical problems*, ed 10, St Louis, 2017, Mosby.

## "FOUR" SCORE NEUROLOGICAL ASSESSMENT SCALE

### Eye Response (E)

| | |
|---|---|
| E4 | Eyelids open or opened, tracking, or blinking to command |
| E3 | Eyelids open but not tracking |
| E2 | Eyelids closed, open to loud voice, not tracking |
| E1 | Eyelids closed, open to pain, not tracking |
| E0 | Eyelids remain closed with pain |

### Motor Response (M)

| | |
|---|---|
| M4 | Thumbs up, fist, or peace sign to command |
| M3 | Localizing to pain |
| M2 | Flexion response to pain |
| M1 | Exterior posturing |
| M0 | No response to pain or generalized myoclonus status epilepticus |

### Brain Stem Reflexes (B)

| | |
|---|---|
| B4 | Pupil and corneal reflexes present |
| B3 | One pupil wide and fixed |
| B2 | Pupil *or* corneal reflexes absent |
| B1 | Pupil *and* corneal reflexes absent |
| B0 | Pupil, corneal, and cough reflexes absent |

### Respiration (R)

| | |
|---|---|
| R4 | Not intubated, regular breathing pattern |
| R3 | Not intubated, Cheyne-Stokes breathing pattern |
| R2 | Not intubated, irregular breathing pattern |
| R1 | Breathes above ventilator rate |
| R0 | Breathes at ventilator rate or has apnea |

From Wijdicks EF, Mamlet WR, et al: Validation of new coma scale: the FOUR Score, *Ann Neurol* 58(4):585, 2005; and Wolf CA, Wijdick EF, et al: Further validation of the FOUR Score coma scale by intensive care nurses, *Mayo Clin Proc* 82(4):435, 2007. Reproduced by permission of Mayo Foundation for Medical Education and Research. All rights reserved.

Clinical Quick Reference

## Fall Risk Factors

The risk of falling becomes greater when a patient becomes ill. Fever, electrolyte imbalance, and dulled mental alertness often contribute to a fall, especially for the elderly patient. General factors that contribute to falls include the following:

- Medications that cause postural hypotension or dizziness; polypharmacy (sedatives, hypnotics, antihypertensives, diuretics, antidepressants, laxatives)
- Muscle weakness from inactivity or illness (stroke)
- Gait alteration resulting from disease or injury; neuropathy in the feet and legs (diabetes)
- Vision problems or dirty eyeglasses
- Balance or gait problem (after stroke or neurologic disorder)
- Alcohol use
- Mental changes: dementia, delirium
- Incontinence and urgency
- Neurologic diseases (stroke, Parkinson disease, multiple sclerosis, etc.)
- Illness and fever
- Severe osteoporosis and spontaneous fracture
- Environmental hazards (e.g., scatter rugs, pets, stairs, slippery floors or showers, small objects on floors, cords in pathways)
- Often, a combination of factors causes a person to fall (Fig. 5.1).

## Fall Risk Assessment Scales

Nursing fall risk assessment, diagnoses, and interventions are based on use of the Morse Fall Scale (MFS) (Morse, 1997; available at: http://www.ahrq.gov/professionals/systems/hospital/fallpxtoolkit/fallpxtk-tool3h.html. The MFS is used widely in acute care settings, both in hospital and long-term care inpatient settings. The MFS requires systematic, reliable assessment of a patient's fall risk factors upon admission, fall, change in status, and discharge or transfer to a new setting. MFS subscales include assessment of:

| | | |
|---|---|---|
| 1. | History of falling; immediate or within 3 months | No = 0<br>Yes = 25 |
| 2. | Secondary diagnosis | No = 0<br>Yes = 15 |
| 3. | Ambulatory aid | None, bed rest, wheelchair, nurse = 0<br>Crutches, cane, walker = 15<br>Furniture = 30 |
| 4. | IV/saline lock | No = 0<br>Yes = 20 |
| 5. | Gait/transferring | Normal, bed rest, immobile = 0<br>Weak = 10<br>Impaired = 20 |
| 6. | Mental status | Oriented to own ability = 0<br>Forgets limitations = 15 |

| Risk Level | MFS Score | Action |
|---|---|---|
| No risk | 0 | None |
| Low risk | <25 | Use Standard Fall Prevention Interventions |
| Moderate risk | 25-45 | Use Standard Fall Prevention Interventions |
| High risk | >45 | Use High Risk Fall Prevention Interventions |

Retrieved from: http://www.ahrq.gov/professionals/systems/hospital/fallpxtoolkit/fallpxtk-tool3h.html

**Fall Risk Assessment**

*Place a check mark in front of the items that apply to the patient.*

General Information

___ Age over 70

___ History of falls*

___ Confusion at times

___ Confused most of the time*

___ Impaired memory or judgment

___ Unable to follow directions*

___ Needs assistance with elimination

___ Visual impairment

___ Feels physically weak*

Medications

___ Receiving central nervous system suppressants (narcotic, sedative, tranquilizer, hypnotic, antidepressant, psychotropic, anticonvulsant)

___ Receiving medication that causes orthostatic hypotension (antihypertensive, diuretic)*

___ Medication that may cause diarrhea (cathartic)

___ Medication that may alter blood glucose levels (insulin, hypoglycemics)

Gait and Balance

___ Poor balance when standing*

___ Balance problems when walking*

___ Swaying, lurching, or slapping gait*

___ Unstable when making turns*

___ Needs assistive device (walker, cane, holds on to furniture)*

Note: A check mark on any starred item indicates a risk for falls. A combination of four or more of the unstarred items indicates a risk for falls.

**FIG. 5.1**    Fall risk assessment. (From Williams P: *Fundamental concepts and skills for nursing*, ed 5, St Louis, 2018, Saunders.)

## Pitting Edema Scale

To assess for pitting edema, depress the skin with your fingertips over the tibia or the medial malleolus for 5 seconds, and then release. Normally there is no edema except during pregnancy or when the person has been standing all day. Check all dependent areas for edema, including the sacrum.

| | |
|---|---|
| 1 + = Trace | Pit is barely seen, 2mm depth |
| 2 + = Mild | Pit is deeper and rebounds within a few seconds, 4mm depth |
| 3 + = Moderate | Deep pit is formed, 6mm depth |
| 4 + = Severe | Deeper pit is formed that may take more than 30 seconds to rebound, 8mm depth |

Adapted from Cooper K, Gosnell K: *Foundations of nursing*, ed 7, St Louis, 2015, Mosby.

Clinical Quick Reference

## Skin Pressure Points

Pressure points (Fig. 5.2) should be examined whenever a patient is repositioned but must be assessed every 2 hours for the immobilized patient.

### RISK FACTORS FOR PRESSURE ULCERS

Consider patients with the following problems as having high risk for skin breakdown and pressure ulcers:

- Immobility (e.g., stroke, paraplegia, quadriplegia, severe trauma, traction)
- Malnutrition and low body weight; hypoalbuminemia
- Dehydration
- Incontinence
- Anemia
- Peripheral vascular disease
- Diabetes mellitus
- Dementia
- Edema
- Dry skin
- Fracture
- Malignancy
- Infection

Various tools may be used to assess the risk for skin breakdown. One such tool commonly used by inpatient facilities is the Braden Scale (Fig. 5.3).

### STAGING PRESSURE ULCERS

The following staging criteria are recommended by the National Pressure Ulcer Advisory Panel and the Agency for Healthcare Research and Quality (AHRQ). Pressure ulcers, once originally staged, should not be *reverse staged*—that is, a stage IV ulcer remains a stage IV until it becomes a *healed stage IV*. Healing is

**FIG. 5.2**   Pressure points.

Braden Scale

## FOR PREDICTING PRESSURE SORE RISK

Patient's Name _____    Evaluator's Name _____    Date of Assessment

| | | | | | Date of Assessment | | |
|---|---|---|---|---|---|---|---|

**SENSORY PERCEPTION**
ability to respond meaningfully to pressure-related discomfort

**1. Completely Limited:** Unresponsive (does not moan, flinch, or grasp) to painful stimuli, due to diminished level of consciousness or sedation
OR
limited ability to feel pain over most of body surface.

**2. Very Limited:** Responds only to painful stimuli. Cannot communicate discomfort except by moaning or restlessness
OR
has a sensory impairment which limits the ability to feel pain or discomfort over 1/2 of body.

**3. Slightly Limited:** Responds to verbal commands, but cannot always communicate discomfort or need to be turned
OR
has some sensory impairment which limits ability to feel pain or discomfort in 1 or 2 extremities.

**4. No Impairment:** Responds to verbal commands. Has no sensory deficit which would limit ability to feel or voice pain or discomfort.

**MOISTURE**
degree to which skin is exposed to moisture

**1. Constantly Moist:** Skin is kept moist almost constantly by perspiration, urine, etc. Dampness is detected every time patient is moved or turned.

**2. Very Moist:** Skin is often, but not always moist. Linen must be changed at least once a shift.

**3. Occasionally Moist:** Skin is occasionally moist, requiring an extra linen change approximately once a day.

**4. Rarely Moist:** Skin is usually dry; linen only requires changing at routine intervals.

**ACTIVITY**
degree of physical activity

**1. Bedfast:** Confined to bed

**2. Chairfast:** Ability to walk severely limited or non-existent. Cannot bear own weight and/or must be assisted into chair or wheelchair.

**3. Walks Occasionally:** Walks occasionally during day, but for very short distances, with or without assistance. Spends majority of each shift in bed or chair.

**4. Walks Frequently:** Walks outside the room at least twice a day and inside room at least once every 2 hours during waking hours.

**MOBILITY**
ability to change and control body position

**1. Completely Immobile:** Does not make even slight changes in body or extremity position without assistance.

**2. Very Limited:** Makes occasional slight changes in body or extremity position but unable to make frequent or significant changes independently.

**3. Slightly Limited:** Makes frequent though slight changes in body or extremity position independently.

**4. No Limitations:** Makes major and frequent changes in position without assistance.

**NUTRITION**
usual food intake pattern

**1. Very Poor:** Never eats a complete meal. Rarely eats more than 1/3 of any food offered. Eats 2 servings or less of protein (meat or dairy products) per day. Takes fluids poorly. Does not take a liquid dietary supplement
OR
is NPO and/or maintained on clear liquids or IV's for more than 5 days.

**2. Probably Inadequate:** Rarely eats a complete meal and generally eats only about 1/2 of any food offered. Protein intake includes only 3 servings of meat or dairy products per day. Occasionally will take a dietary supplement
OR
receives less than optimum amount of liquid diet or tube feeding.

**3. Adequate:** Eats over half of most meals. Eats a total of 4 servings of protein (meat, dairy products) each day. Occasionally will refuse a meal, but will usually take a supplement if offered
OR
is on a tube feeding or TPN regimen that probably meets most of nutritional needs.

**4. Excellent:** Eats most of every meal. Never refuses a meal. Usually eats a total of 4 or more servings of meat and dairy products. Occasionally eats between meals. Does not require supplementation.

**FRICTION AND SHEAR**

**1. Problem:** Requires moderate to maximum assistance in moving. Complete lifting without sliding against sheets is impossible. Frequently slides down in bed or chair, requiring frequent repositioning with maximum assistance. Spasticity, contractures or agitation leads to almost constant friction.

**2. Potential Problem:** Moves feebly or requires minimum assistance. During a move, skin probably slides to some extent against sheets, chair, restraints, or other devices. Maintains relatively good position in chair or bed most of the time but occasionally slides down.

**3. No Apparent Problem:** Moves in bed and in chair independently and has sufficient muscle strength to lift up completely during move. Maintains good position in bed or chair at all times.

Total Score _____

Key: At risk, 15–18; Moderate risk, 13–14; High risk, 10–12; Severe risk, 9.

**FIG. 5.3**  Braden Scale for Predicting Pressure Sore Risk. (Copyright 1988, Barbara Braden and Nancy Bergstrom. Reprinted with permission.)

documented by improvement in wound size, depth, amount of necrotic tissue, and amount of exudate. Eschar must be débrided before proper staging can occur.

| | |
|---|---|
| Suspected deep tissue injury | Localized discolored intact skin that is maroon or purple or a blood-filled blister resulting from damage to underlying soft tissue from pressure or shear. The area may be painful, firm, mushy, boggy, warmer, or cooler when compared with adjacent tissue. |
| Stage I | An area of red, deep pink, or mottled skin that does not blanch with fingertip pressure. In people with darker skin, discoloration of the skin, warmth, edema, or induration may be signs of a stage I pressure ulcer. |
| Stage II | Partial-thickness skin loss involving epidermis, dermis, or both. May appear as an abrasion, a blister, or a shallow crater. Area around damaged skin may feel warmer. |
| Stage III | Full-thickness skin loss that looks like a deep crater and may extend to the fascia. Subcutaneous tissue is damaged or necrotic. Bacterial infection of the ulcer is common and causes drainage from the ulcer. There may be damage to the surrounding tissue. |
| Stage IV | Full-thickness skin loss with extensive tissue necrosis, or damage to muscle, bone, or supporting structures (e.g., tendon, joint capsule). Undermining and sinus tracts (tunnels) may also be present. Infection is usually widespread. The ulcer may appear dry and black, with a buildup of tough, necrotic tissue (eschar), or it can appear wet and oozing. |
| Unstageable | Loss of full thickness of tissue. The base of the ulcer is covered by eschar (tan, brown, or black) in the wound bed, or the base of the ulcer contains slough (yellow, tan, gray, green, or brown). |

Adapted from Williams P: *Fundamental concepts and skills for nursing*, ed 5, St Louis, 2018, Saunders.

## Substance Abuse Screening—CAGE

**C**ut down: "Have you ever thought you should **cut down** on your drinking or drug use?"

**A**nnoyed: "Have people **annoyed** you by criticizing your drinking or drug use?"

**G**uilty: "Have you felt bad or **guilty** about your drinking or drug use?"

**E**ye-opener: "Have you ever had a drink or used drugs first thing in the morning to steady your nerves or to get rid of a hangover **(eye-opener)**?"

*Answering yes to any of these questions indicates that the patient may have a substance abuse problem.*

Adapted from *Mosby's PDQ for LPN*, ed 4, St Louis, 2017, Mosby.

## Erikson's Stages of Development

Nursing students are often asked to place the patient within one of Erikson's stages of development by listing some behaviors to verify the correct stage. The following chart provides a listing of sample behaviors that are appropriate for each stage:

| Verbal Behaviors | Nonverbal Behaviors |
|---|---|
| **Trust vs. Mistrust (Birth to 18 Months)** | |
| ***Trust*** | |
| "I believe you." "I know I can tell you…" "You will help me." "You are my friend." | Asking for help with the expectation of receiving it. Accepting help from others comfortably. Sharing time, opinions, emotions, and experiences. |

## Erikson's Stages of Development—cont'd

| Verbal Behaviors | Nonverbal Behaviors |
|---|---|

### Mistrust

"I am afraid of you."
"I can't tell you about anything."
"You cheat."

Inability to accept help. Confining conversation to superficialities. Rigidly controlling behavior so that only that which is socially approved is exhibited. Refusal to share time, experiences, opinions, and emotions.

### Autonomy vs. Shame and Doubt (1½ to 3 Years)

#### Autonomy

"I will."
"I won't."
"Okay, I'll do it myself."
"This is my opinion."
"I can wait."

Tries to dress self or perform other tasks on own. Accepting group rules but able to express dissent when it is felt. Accepting leadership role when it is appropriate. Expressing own opinion. Accepting postponement of wish gratification easily. Ability to cooperate. Demonstrates some self-control.

#### Shame and Doubt

"My opinion doesn't count."
"I never know the answers."
"I don't want to hear what you have to say."
"I must be right."
"I should do that."

Overly concerned with being clean. Not maintaining own opinion when opposed. Failing to express needs. Maintaining own opinion despite adequate proof to the contrary. Lacks self-control. Unable to wait; hoarding; soiling. Being vindictive.

### Initiative vs. Guilt (3 to 6 Years)

#### Initiative

"Let me try."
"What is it? How does it work?"
"Where does that road go?"
"May I wash my hair?"

Exploring. Starting new projects with eagerness. Expressing curiosity. Being original. Ability to evaluate own behavior. Brushes teeth without being told.

#### Guilt

"I'm afraid to do that."
"You go first, and I will follow."
"I'm ashamed to make a mistake."

Imitating others rather than developing ideas independently. Expressing a great deal of embarrassment over a small mistake. Always taking the blame.

### Industry vs. Inferiority (7 to 10 Years)

#### Industry

"I'm working on this. When it is done, I will start on that."
"I like to be busy."
"Group projects are fun."
"I'm going to do my homework now."

Completing a task once it is started. Working well with others. Using time effectively. Feelings of competence. Good self-esteem.

#### Inferiority

"I can't work with other people."
"I have a lot of things going but nothing finished."
"I don't think I can do it."

Not completing any set tasks. Not contributing to the work of the group. Not organizing work. Avoids responsibility.

Clinical Quick Reference

Continued

# Erikson's Stages of Development—cont'd

| Verbal Behaviors | Nonverbal Behaviors |
|---|---|

## Identity vs. Role Diffusion (10 to 17 Years)

### Identity

"I'm going to be a nurse."
"I believe in these principles."
"I think mothers should do this, and fathers should do that."
"I know where I'm going."
"I feel good about myself."

Establishing relationships with the same sex and then with the opposite sex. Planning realistically for the future. Reexamining values. Asserting independence. Trying various things.

### Role Diffusion

"I don't know who I am."
"Where am I going?"
"Is it better to be male or female?"
"I don't know what I mean."

Failing to differentiate roles or goals in life. Failing to assume responsibility for directing own behavior. Imitating others indiscriminately. Accepting the values of others without question.

## Intimacy vs. Isolation (18 to 40 Years)

### Intimacy

"We are very close friends."
"I love Dan."
"My family is very close."
"I have lots of good friends."

Establishing a close and intense relationship with another person. Acting out and accepting appropriate sexual behavior as desirable. Maintaining a marital or other monogamous relationship.

### Isolation

"I'm a loner."
"I don't need anyone."
"I don't care about anyone."
"I'm very lonely."

Remaining alone. Not seeking out others for companionship or help. Avoiding sex role by remaining nondescript in mannerisms and dress.

## Generativity vs. Stagnation (40 to 65 Years)

### Generativity

"John and I have agreed to have two children."
"He has his work and I have mine…together we make a team."
"I am raising three children."
"I am employed at…"
"I love to sew."

Productive. Maintaining employment. Parenting. Accepting interdependence. Guiding others. Creative. Community or church leadership. Completes creative endeavors; has hobbies. Performs own self-care and takes responsibility for own health.

### Stagnation

"I can't hold a job."
"I don't want to learn about it."
"I haven't time to volunteer."
"You do it; I'm going out."
"That's too bad, but it isn't my problem."

Not listening to others because of need to talk about oneself. Constantly losing employment. Showing concern only for oneself despite the needs of others. Self-absorption. Always finds excuses. Refuses to learn self-care.

## Integrity vs. Despair (65 Years to Death)

### Integrity

"Life has been very good to me."
"I can't do the things I once did, but I enjoy other things."
"I enjoy discussing current events."
"I read the newspaper every day."
"I love watching the birds at the feeder."
"I enjoy seeing my children and my grandchildren."

Using past experiences to guide others. Accepting new ideas. Accepting limitations. Maintaining productivity in some area. Exploring philosophy of living and dying. Enjoying some aspect of things as they are. Actively participating in own care as much as able.

## Erikson's Stages of Development—cont'd

| Verbal Behaviors | Nonverbal Behaviors |
|---|---|
| ***Despair*** | |
| "I am no use to anyone."<br>"Everyone is gone…my family, my friends."<br>"What is the use of living; I can't do anything."<br>"Everything I did is gone now. Why did this happen?"<br>"These new ways are no good." | Crying; being apathetic and listless. Not developing any new interests beyond a few routine activities. Developing no new relationships. Not accepting changes. Limiting interpersonal contacts. Demanding unnecessary help and attention. Remaining in pajamas and robe all the time. |

## Piaget's Cognitive Developmental Stages

| Stage | Characterized By |
|---|---|
| Sensorimotor<br>Birth to 2 years | Begins to differentiate self from others and objects. Recognizes self as agent of action and starts acting intentionally with simple repetitive actions; shakes a rattle to make noise.<br>Object permanence is achieved; understands that things still exist even when no longer within range of vision. Egocentric. |
| Preoperational<br>2 to 7 years | Learns to use language; represents objects with images and words (uses symbols while thinking).<br>Still egocentric in thinking; has difficulty in taking the viewpoint of others. Thinks others see the world as he/she does. |
| Concrete operational<br>7 to 11 years | Reasoning and thought become logical, but limited to own experience.<br>Understands cause and effect.<br>Can classify objects according to several features and has ability to order them in series such as by size.<br>By age 6 achieves conservation of number; by age 7, conservation of mass; and by age 9, conservation of weight. |
| Formal operational<br>11 years and up | Acquires ability to develop abstract concepts for self.<br>Oriented to problem solving.<br>Grows to be concerned with the hypothetical, the future, and ideological matters. |

Data from Leifer G: *Introduction to maternity & pediatric nursing*, ed 7, St Louis, 2015, Mosby; Potter PA, et al: *Basic nursing*, ed 7, St Louis, 2012, Mosby; Atherton JS: *Learning and teaching: Piaget's developmental theory*. http://www.learningandteaching.info/learning/piaget.htm, 2011.

## Child Abuse and Neglect

One sign by itself does not necessarily indicate a problem, but be alert for the following signs, which call for a more in-depth assessment for possible abuse:
* Suspicious bruises, lacerations, burns, fractures, or head injury
* Welts, bite marks, or clumps of hair loss
* Abdominal injury with suspicious history
* Repeated or multiple fractures without an adequate history of precipitating events
* Unkempt or dirty appearance, inappropriate clothing for the weather
* Failure to thrive
* Wariness or clinging to adults who are strangers or getting upset when another child cries
* Fearfulness of parents or other adults
* A sophisticated knowledge of sexual activities

Clinical Quick Reference

- Promiscuity and defiance of authority
- Adult behavior such as belittling the child, constantly blaming the child, repeatedly embarrassing the child, or withholding love and affection from the child
  Remember that some odd skin markings can be from a cultural practice such as "coining," in which a coin is rubbed over the skin to help relieve illness. This practice is not abuse. If signs of abuse are definite, they must be reported.

## Elder Abuse and Neglect

One sign alone does not necessarily indicate abuse, but some telltale signs that there could be a problem are as follows:

- Bruises, black eyes, lacerations, puncture wounds, pressure marks, broken bones, burns, abrasions
- Signs of marks from restraints
- Untreated injuries in various stages of healing
- Sprains, dislocations, or internal injuries
- Pressure ulcers, poor hygiene, or unattended medical needs
- Bruises around the genital area or breasts
- Unusual weight loss in combination with other signs
- Unkempt; inappropriate dress or hygiene
- Unusual fear exhibited
- An unexplained extreme withdrawal from usual activities
- Abrupt change in behavior
- A sudden change in alertness and indications of depression (may indicate emotional abuse)
- Inappropriate clothing for the weather
- Dehydration and/or malnutrition
- Broken eyeglasses
- Medication overdose or underutilization
- Caregiver refusal to allow visitors to see elderly person alone
- Sudden changes in financial situation
- Caregiver or spouse behavior such as belittling or threats
- Strained or tense relationships, frequent arguments with the caregiver or spouse

# ■ PAIN

## The Joint Commission (TJC) Pain Standards

The following is a summary of the standards for pain assessment for all patients in any setting from TJC:

1. Patients have the right to appropriate assessment and management of pain.
2. Pain will be assessed in all patients in a timely and recurring manner.
3. Policies and procedures must support safe medication prescription or ordering.
4. Patients must be educated, as appropriate, about pain and managing pain as part of treatment.
5. The discharge process will provide for continuing pain care based on the patient's assessed needs at the time of discharge.
6. Organizations will collect data to monitor their performance, addressing the following areas:
   - Appropriate pain assessment and management
   - Effective pain treatment or referral for treatment
   - Timely assessment and reassessment of pain, including the nature and intensity
   - Patient involvement in making decisions about pain management

- Education for staff and patients regarding the following:
  - The importance of effective pain management
  - Pain management as a part of total treatment
  - Continuing pain care after discharge
  - Documentation of pain assessments, treatments, and evaluation of effectiveness
  - Staff competency in pain assessment and management

Pain is considered the fifth vital sign and should be assessed whenever vital signs are taken. After assessment, documentation of the findings must be completed. Numerous pain assessment tools are available. Use the scale that is designated in the pain assessment procedure for your agency.

## Focused Assessment for the Patient with Pain

### LOCATION
- Where is your pain?
- Does the pain radiate (e.g., into arms, back, down legs, etc.)?

### CHARACTERISTICS
- Describe your pain.
- What words would describe your pain (e.g., aching, burning, gnawing, sharp, dull, continuous, intermittent)?

### QUANTITY
- Use a pain scale (e.g., numeric, descriptive).

### PATTERN
- When did the pain start?
- Did the pain begin during or after an activity or eating?
- Did the pain start suddenly?
- Has the pain increased over time?

### ASSOCIATED FACTORS
- Have you had other symptoms (e.g., shortness of breath, nausea, vomiting, palpitations, or sweating)?

### ALLEVIATING FACTORS
- What have you used to relieve the pain (e.g., over-the-counter [OTC] medications, position change)?
- Did the measures that you tried provide relief?

### AGGRAVATING FACTORS
- What (if anything) makes the pain worse?

---

Modified from deWit SC, Stromberg H, Dallred C: *Medical-surgical nursing: concepts and practice*, ed 3, St Louis, 2016, Saunders.

## Pain Rating Scales

### NUMERIC PAIN SCALE
The patient rates the pain on a scale of 0 to 10, with 0 being no pain and 10 being unbearable pain.

Clinical Quick Reference

## UNIVERSAL PAIN ASSESSMENT

### UNIVERSAL PAIN ASSESSMENT TOOL

This pain assessment tool is intended to help patient care providers assess pain according to individual patient needs. Explain and use 0–10 Scale for patient self-assessment. Use the faces or behavioral observations to interpret expressed pain when patient cannot communicate his/her pain intensity.

| | 0 No pain | 1–2 | 3–4 | 5–6 | 7–8 | 9–10 |
|---|---|---|---|---|---|---|
| WONG-BAKER FACIAL GRIMACE SCALE | 0 | 1–2 | 3–4 | 5–6 | 7–8 | 9–10 |
| | | MILD | MODERATE | | SEVERE | |
| ACTIVITY TOLERANCE SCALE | NO PAIN | CAN BE IGNORED | INTERFERES WITH TASKS | INTERFERES WITH CONCENTRATION | INTERFERES WITH BASIC NEEDS | BEDREST REQUIRED |
| SPANISH | NADA DE DOLOR | UN POQUITO DE DOLOR | UN DOLOR LEVE | DOLOR FUERTE | DOLOR DEMASIADO FUERTE | UN DOLOR INSOPORTABLE |
| FRENCH | AUCUNE DOULEUR | LÉGÈRE DOULEUR | DOULEUR MODÉRÈE | FORTE DOULEUR | TRÈS FORTE DOULEUR | DOULEUR EXTREME |
| GERMAN | KEINE SCHMERZEN | LEICHTE SCHMERZEN | MÄSSIGE SCHMERZEN | STARKE SCHMERZEN | SEHR STARKE SCHMERZEN | EXTREME SCHMERZEN |
| JAPANESE | 痛みなし | 軽い痛み | 中程度の痛み | ひどい痛み | 非常にひどい痛み | 最悪の痛み |
| TAGALOG | HINDI MASAKIT | KAUNTIG SAKIT | MEDYO MASAKIT | TALAGANG MASAKIT | MASAKITNA MASAKIT | PINAKAMASAKIT |
| HINDI | DARDNAHI HAI | BAHUT KAM | HILNE SE TAKLEF HOTI HAI | SOCH NAHIN SAKTE | KUCH NAHIN KAR SAKTE | DARD BAHUT HAI |

Reprinted with permission from UCLA Department of Anesthesiology, David Geffen School of Medicine at UCLA: The Wong-Baker FACES Rating Scale; adapted from Hockenberry MJ, Wilson D: *Wong's nursing care of infants and children*, ed 10, St Louis, 2015, Mosby.

## DESCRIPTIVE WORD RATING SCALE

Chart rating over scale (e.g., 3/5).

| 0 | 1 | 2 | 3 | 4 | 5 |
|---|---|---|---|---|---|
| No pain | Mild | Discomforting | Distressing | Horrible | Excruciating |

## VISUAL ANALOG SCALE (VAS)

Have the patient indicate the degree of pain by marking the line below:

No pain at all _____ Greatest pain possible

## VERBAL DESCRIPTOR SCALE (VDS)

Have the patient check the best descriptor of his or her pain at this moment (may read to the resident):

_____ absent
_____ minimal
_____ mild
_____ moderate
_____ fairly severe

_____ severe
_____ very severe
_____ extremely severe
_____ exquisite
_____ unbearable

# NEONATAL/INFANT PAIN SCALE (NIPS)

**Pain Assessment Tools**

**Neonatal/Infant Pain Scale (NIPS)**

(Recommended for children less than 1 year old)—A score greater than 3 indicates pain

| Pain Assessment | | Score |
|---|---|---|
| **Facial Expression**<br>0 – Relaxed muscles<br>1 – Grimace | Restful face, neutral expression<br>Tight facial muscles; furrowed brow, chin, jaw (negative facial expression—nose, mouth and brow) | |
| **Cry**<br>0 – No Cry<br>1 – Whimper<br>2 – Vigorous Cry | Quiet, not crying<br>Mild moaning, intermittent<br>Loud scream; rising, shrill, continuous (Note: Silent cry may be scored if baby is intubated as evidenced by obvious mouth and facial movement) | |
| **Breathing Patterns**<br>0 – Relaxed<br>1 – Change in Breathing | Usual pattern for this infant<br>Indrawing, irregular, faster than usual; gagging; breath holding | |
| **Arms**<br>0 – Relaxed/Restrained<br>1 – Flexed/Extended | No muscular rigidity; occasional random movements of arms<br>Tense, straight legs; rigid and/or rapid extension, flexion | |
| **Legs**<br>0 – Relaxed/Restrained<br>1 – Flexed/Extended | No muscular rigidity; occasional random leg movement<br>Tense, straight legs; rigid and/or rapid extension, flexion | |
| **State of Arousal**<br>0 – Sleeping/Awake<br>1 – Fussy | Quiet, peaceful, sleeping or alert, random leg movement<br>Alert, restless, and thrashing | |

From Lawrence J, Alcock D, McGrath P, et al: The development of a tool to assess neonatal pain, *Neonatal Network* 12(6):59-66, 1993. Reprinted with permission from Children's Hospital of Eastern Ontario, Ottawa, Ontario, Canada.

Clinical Quick Reference

## REVISED FLACC SCALE

| | 0 | 1 | 2 |
|---|---|---|---|
| **F**—Face | No particular expression or smile | Occasional grimace or frown, withdrawn, disinterested<br>*Appears sad or worried* | Frequent-to-constant frown, clenched jaw, quivering chin<br>*Distress-looking face: expression of fright or panic* |
| **L**—Legs | Normal position or relaxed | Uneasy, restless, tense<br>*Occasional tremors* | Kicking or legs drawn up<br>*Marked increase in spasticity, constant tremors or jerking* |
| **A**—Activity | Lying quietly, normal position, moves easily | Squirming, shifting back and forth, tense<br>*Mildly agitated (e.g., head back and forth, aggression); shallow, splinting respirations; intermittent sighs* | Arched, rigid, or jerking<br>*Severe agitation, head banging, shivering (not rigors); breath-holding, gasping or sharp intake of breath; severe splinting* |
| **C**—Cry | No crying (awake or asleep) | Moans or whimpers, occasional complaint<br>*Occasional verbal outburst or grunt* | Crying steadily, screams or sobs, frequent complaints<br>*Repeated outbursts, constant grunting* |
| **C**—Consolability | Content, relaxed | Reassured by occasional touching, hugging, or talking to; distractible | Difficult to console or comfort<br>*Pushing away caregiver, resisting care or comfort measures* |

Each of the five categories is scored from 0-2, which results in a total score between 0 and 10.

**Patients who are awake:** Observe for at least 1-2 minutes. Observe legs and body uncovered. Reposition patient or observe activity, assess body for tenseness and tone. Initiate consoling interventions if needed.

**Patients who are asleep:** Observe for at least 2 minutes or longer. Observe body and legs uncovered. If possible reposition the patient. Touch the body and assess for tenseness and tone.

**The revised FLACC** can be used for all nonverbal children. The additional descriptors (in bold) are descriptors validated in children with cognitive impairment. The nurse can review with parents the descriptors within each category. Ask them if there are additional behaviors that are better indicators of pain in their child. Add these behaviors to the tool in the appropriate category.

Copyright © 2002, The Regents of the University of Michigan. From Malviya S, Voepel-Lewis T, Burke CN, et al: The revised FLACC observational pain tool: Improved reliability and validity for pain assessment in children with cognitive impairment. *Pediatr Anesthesia* 16:258-265, 2006.

## FLACC BEHAVIORAL PAIN SCALE
### F—Face
Score 0 points if patient has a relaxed face, eye contact, and interest in
surroundings
Score 1 point if patient has a worried look to face, with eyebrows lowered, eyes
partially closed, cheeks raised, mouth pursed
Score 2 points if patient has deep furrows in the forehead, with closed eyes, open
mouth, and deep lines around nose/lips

### L—Legs
Score 0 points if patient has usual tone and motion to limbs (legs and arms)
Score 1 point if patient has increased tone, rigidity, tense, intermittent flexion/
extension of limbs
Score 2 points if patient has hypertonicity, legs pulled tight, exaggerated flexion/
extension of limbs, tremors

### A—Activity
Score 0 points if patient moves easily and freely, normal activity/restrictions
Score 1 point if patient shifts positions, hesitant to move, guarding, tense torso,
pressure on body part
Score 2 points if patient is in fixed position, rocking, side-to-side head movement,
rubbing body part

### C—Cry
Score 0 points if patient has no cry/moan awake or asleep
Score 1 point if patient has occasional moans, cries, whimpers, sighs
Score 2 points if patient has frequent/continuous moans, cries, grunts

### C—Consolability
Score 0 points if patient is calm and does not require consoling
Score 1 point if patient responds to comfort by touch or talk in ½-1 minute
Score 2 points if patient requires constant consoling or is unconsoled after an
extended time
Whenever feasible, behavioral measurement of pain should be used in
conjunction with self-report. When self-report is not possible, interpretation of pain behaviors and decision making regarding treatment of pain
requires careful consideration of the context in which the pain behaviors were
observed.
Each category is scored on the 0-2 scale, which results in a total score of 0-10.

### Assessment of Behavioral Score
0 = Relaxed and comfortable
1-3 = Mild discomfort
4-6 = Moderate pain
7-10 = Severe discomfort/pain

Copyright 2002, The Regents of the University of Michigan. From Merkel S, Voepel-Lewis T,
Shayevitz J, Malviya S: The FLACC: A behavioral scale for scoring postoperative pain in
young children. *Pediatr Nursing* 23:293-297, 1997.

## MEMORY DEVICE FOR ASSESSMENT OF PAIN: PQRST

| Factor | Questions to Ask |
|---|---|
| **P**—Precipitating events | What events or factors (e.g., activity, exercise, resting) precipitated the pain or discomfort? |
| **Q**—Quality of pain or discomfort | What does the pain or discomfort feel like (e.g., dull, aching, sharp, tight)? |
| **R**—Radiation of pain | Where is the pain located? Where does the pain radiate to (e.g., back, arms, jaw, teeth, shoulder, elbow)? |
| **S**—Severity of pain | On a scale of 0 to 10, with 10 being the most severe pain, how would you rate the pain or discomfort? |
| **T**—Timing | When did the pain or discomfort begin? Has the pain changed since that time? Have you had pain like this before? |

This memory device may be used for pain in other locations as well.

Adapted from Lewis SM, Bucher L, Heitkemper MM, et al: *Medical-surgical nursing: assessment and management of clinical problems*, ed 10, St Louis, 2017, Mosby.

## MEASURES TO RELIEVE PAIN AND DISCOMFORT
- Relieve extraneous sensory input by providing a quiet, tidy environment.
- Administer pain medication promptly; reassess patient for pain level in 30 minutes (depending on route) and at the time the next dose should be given.
- Advise patient to ask for pain medication before pain becomes severe; medication is more effective if given before the onset of severe pain.
- Provide distraction with reading material, a TV program, pleasant music, a game, or conversation.
- Offer a massage.
- Teach relaxation exercises.
- Assist with a pleasant imagery exercise.
- Straighten bed linens and position for comfort.
- Seek to reduce anxieties if possible.
- Encourage verbalization of fears.
- Provide other analgesics between narcotic doses, if ordered.
- Encourage use of heat or cold treatments as ordered.
- Determine whether pain medication ordered is effective; if not, request an order change from the physician.
- Remember that just because a patient may go to sleep, it does not mean that the pain medication is not needed.

## MNEMONIC FOR CHARTING PAIN ASSESSMENT: OLDCART
- **O**nset
- **L**ocation
- **D**uration
- **C**haracteristics
- **A**ggravating factors
- **R**elieving factors
- **T**reatments

## Equianalgesic Doses of Opioids

| Drug and Route* | Equianalgesic Dose (mg)† | TIME COURSE OF ANALGESIC EFFECTS | | |
|---|---|---|---|---|
| | | Onset (min) | Peak (min) | Duration (hr) |
| **Codeine** | | | | |
| PO | 200 | 30-45 | 60-120 | 4-6 |
| IM | 130 | 10-30 | 30-60 | 4-6 |
| Subcut | 130 | 10-30 | 30-60 | 4-6 |
| **Hydrocodone** | | | | |
| PO | 30 | 10-30 | 30-60 | 4-6 |
| **Hydromorphone** | | | | |
| PO | 7.5 | 30 | 90-120 | 4 |
| IM | 1.5 | 15 | 30-60 | 4-5 |
| IV | 1.5 | 10-15 | 15-30 | 2-3 |
| Subcut | 1.5 | 15 | 30-90 | 4 |
| **Levorphanol** | | | | |
| PO | 4 | 10-60 | 90-120 | 6-8 |
| IM | 2 | — | 60 | 6-8 |
| IV | 2 | — | Within 20 | 6-8 |
| Subcut | 2 | — | 60-90 | 6-8 |
| **Methadone** | | | | |
| PO | 20 | 30-60 | 90-120 | 6-8 |
| IM | 10 | 10-20 | 60-120 | 4-5 |
| IV | 10 | — | 15-30 | 3-4‡ |
| **Morphine** | | | | |
| PO | 30 | — | 60-120 | 3-5 |
| IM | 10 | 10-30 | 30-60 | 3-5 |
| IV | 10 | — | 20 | 3-5 |
| Subcut | 10 | 10-30 | 50-90 | 3-5 |
| Epidural | — | 15-60 | — | Up to 24 |
| Intrathecal | — | 15-60 | — | Up to 24 |
| **Oxycodone** | | | | |
| PO | 10 | 15-30 | 60 | 3-6§ |
| **Oxymorphone** | | | | |
| IM | 1 | 10-15 | 30-90 | 4-6 |
| IV | 1 | 5-10 | 15-30 | 3-4 |
| Subcut | 1 | 10-20 | — | 4-6 |
| Rectal | 10 | 15-30 | 120 | 3-6 |

Use of meperidine is not recommended.

*Intramuscular (IM) administration should be avoided whenever possible. IV, Intravenous; PO, by mouth; Subcut, subcutaneous.

†Dose in milligrams that produces a degree of analgesia equivalent to that produced by a 10-mg IM dose of morphine.

‡With repeated doses, methadone's duration of action may increase up to 48 hours.

§Effects of extended-release formulations may persist for 8 to 12 hours.

Adapted from Hodgson BB, Kizior RJ: *Saunders nursing drug handbook 2017*, St Louis, 2017, Elsevier.

## ■ BASIC NURSING CARE

### Routine Observation of Chest Tubes

- Assess respiratory status.
- Assess for pain and discomfort; medicate as needed.
- Encourage patient to cough and deep-breathe.
- Patient should be in Fowler or high-Fowler position.
- Observe occlusive dressing over insertion site and surrounding skin. Palpate area to assess for crepitus.
- Observe tubing for kinks or obstructions; all connections should be intact and taped.
- Chest drainage collection unit should be below level of chest and upright.
- Add sterile water as needed to water-seal and/or suction control chamber.
- Observe the type and amount of drainage (expect less than 50 to 200 mL/hr dark red blood immediately after surgery; amount of drainage should decrease with time).
- Mark the level of drainage for each shift on the drainage unit.
- Observe for and expect fluctuation in water-seal chamber with respirations.
- No fluctuation suggests a blockage within the system.
- Bubbling in the water-seal chamber may be initially observed as air is leaving the chest. As the pneumothorax resolves, no bubbling should be observed in the water-seal chamber.

### Other Tips for Chest Tube Care

- If wall suction is applied, increase suction only until slight bubbling is seen in the suction control chamber. Increases in wall suction will not cause changes in suction pressure to the chest. Vigorous bubbling will cause evaporation of the water, and changes in the water level WILL change the chest wall suction.
- The drainage collection system is never emptied; replace the entire unit as needed.
- If the wall suction is temporarily disconnected, the water seal remains intact; however, if the system accidentally breaks or tubing becomes disconnected, reestablish the water seal by temporarily placing the distal end of tubing in a container of sterile water. Do not clamp the chest tube.

### Assisting the Patient to Urinate

With the patient positioned for urination:
- Run water in a nearby sink.
- Have a female patient blow through a straw into a glass of water.
- Assist a male patient to stand at the bedside (with a physician's order).
- Allow privacy if patient can be left alone.
- Gently, but firmly, use Credé movements over the bladder (massage from top of bladder to bottom by rocking the palm of the hand over it).
- Place patient in a warm sitz bath (with physician's order). Encourage to void into the sitz bath. Cleanse perineum afterward.
- Pour warm water over the perineum with patient attempting to void. Place the patient's hand in a bowl or pan of warm water.
- Encourage patient to breathe deep and relax; ask patient to visualize running water in a peaceful place.

### Relieving Flatulence (Gas)

- Have the patient ambulate in an upright position as much as possible.
- Seek an order for simethicone medication to decrease gas formation.
- Have the patient avoid carbonated beverages, beverages containing ice, and gas-forming foods.
- Have the patient avoid drinking through a straw (it increases the swallowing of air, which causes gas).
- Use abdominal massage if not contraindicated; massage with a circular motion over the large intestine, moving in the direction that intestinal contents travel. Massage encourages gas to move down the intestinal tract.
- Use measures to stimulate a bowel movement, such as warm water with lemon juice orally, a rectal suppository (if ordered), or measures that usually work for the particular patient.
- If discomfort is severe, ask the physician whether the patient can be placed in Trendelenburg position for short periods to encourage gas to move out of the intestine. (With the intestine and rectum higher than the stomach and head, the gas will move up and out.)

## ■ EMERGENCIES AND CRITICAL CARE

### Nursing Actions in Case of Fire—RACE & PASS

**R**escue any patients in immediate danger by removing them from the area.
**A**ctivate the fire alarm system, and notify the telephone operator.
**C**ontain the fire by closing doors and any open windows.
**E**xtinguish the flames with an appropriate fire extinguisher or **E**vacuate if told to do so.

#### For fire extinguisher use:

**P**ull the lock pin out
**A**im the nozzle at the base of the flames
**S**queeze the handles together
**S**weep from side to side at the base of the flames

### Calling a Rapid Response

If immediate help is needed and the patient is breathing and has a pulse, activate the rapid response team. Usually an advanced practice nurse and respiratory therapist at minimum are part of the team. They can help assess and manage the patient. Protocols allow the response team to initiate some treatments and tests before the arrival of a physician.

### Calling a "Code"

If the patient does not respond to your verbal call, follow basic cardiopulmonary resuscitation (CPR) guidelines. Turn on the call light, shout (if patient is in the bathroom, activate the bathroom call bell), or press the code button on the room wall, or use the phone to call in a code and alert the code team as you begin to do the following:

- Feel for a carotid pulse in an adult or a brachial pulse in an infant, while observing for signs of breathing.
- Begin rescue breathing if pulse is present but the patient is not breathing.
- Breaths are given at a rate of 10-12 per minute using a bag-valve-mask or barrier device.
- Begin CPR (if patient is pulseless), and continue until relieved.
- Give chest compressions at a rate of at least 100 compressions per minute.
- Give ventilations at a rate of 30 compressions and then 2 ventilations.

## Evaluating an ECG Rhythm Strip

When working with patients on telemetry or in the emergency department, you need to be able to do a basic evaluation of an electrocardiographic (ECG) tracing (Fig. 5.4). The following steps provide the needed data regarding the rate, rhythm, P-R interval, duration of the QRS complex, and whether irregular beats are present:

- Obtain a 6-second strip (one with at least 10 large graph squares).
- Calculate the heart rate. Count the number of R waves and multiply by 10.
- Determine if rate is regular or irregular. Measure with calipers from R wave to R wave throughout the tracing to determine whether the rate is regular. Are there premature QRS complexes? Do all the QRS complexes look the same?
- Is there a P wave in front of every QRS complex? (If not, this finding is significant.)
- Measure the P-R interval. Is it normal (0.12 to 0.20 sec)? Does it vary?
- Measure the QRS duration. Is it normal (≥0.12 sec)? Measurement of the Q-T interval is also important in monitoring drug effects.
- Fig. 5.5 shows the results of an analysis of a normal sinus rhythm.

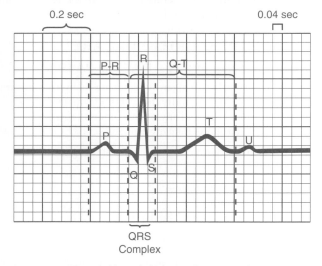

**FIG. 5.4**    Normal electrocardiogram tracing.

1. Rate between 60-100 bpm and regular.
2. P wave precedes each QRS complex; P-R interval between 0.12-0.20 sec (3-5 small squares).
3. QRS duration less than or equal to 0.12 sec (3 small squares).
4. QRS complexes have essentially the same shape.

**FIG. 5.5**    Interpreting an electrocardiogram. (From Lewis SM, Bucher L, Heitkemper MM, et al: *Medical-surgical nursing: assessment and management of clinical problems*, ed 10, St Louis, 2017, Mosby.)

## Telemetry Monitoring

When the patient is started on cardiac telemetry monitoring, one of two leads is most commonly used, either a lead II or a lead $V_1$. Three- and five-electrode systems are the most common. To monitor $V_1$ in a three-lead system, a modified chest lead ($MCL_1$) is obtained. In a five-lead system the monitor designates which electrode is identified as the positive, the negative, and the ground. With the chest electrode placed appropriately, a $V_1$ lead can be obtained. (Fig. 5.6). **Check your hospital's procedure guide.**

## Care and Observation During a Seizure

- Assist the patient to a lying position, move objects out of the way, and loosen any tight clothing.
- Do not restrain the patient.
- Place something soft under the head, if possible, such as a pillow, folded towel, or piece of clothing, if the patient is on a hard surface.
- Gently turn the head to the side to prevent aspiration of saliva.
- Do not force anything into the mouth.
- Note the times that the seizure begins and ends.
- Note the progression of movements because this is important information for the physician.
- Call for assistance, but stay with the patient.

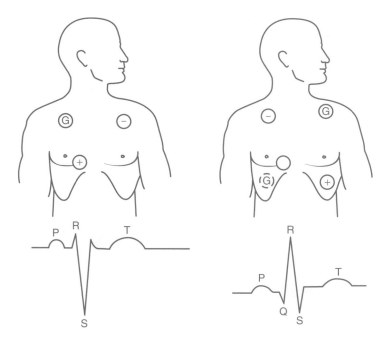

Placement of $MCL_1$ electrodes          Placement of lead II electrodes

**FIG. 5.6**  Placement of most commonly used telemetry leads. (Adapted from Black JM, Hawks JH: *Medical-surgical nursing: clinical management for positive outcomes*, ed 8, Philadelphia, 2009, Saunders.)

Clinical Quick Reference

- Remember that respirations are sometimes irregular or cease for a short period during a seizure.
- Note if the patient becomes incontinent.
- Provide privacy if possible.
- Reassure the patient that you are there.
- After the seizure is over, reorient the patient, and tell him or her that a seizure has occurred.
- Record in detail all observations of the seizure.

## ■ MEASUREMENTS AND CONVERSIONS

### Temperature

Convert Celsius readings to Fahrenheit by multiplying the Celsius reading by 1.8 and adding 32:

$$F = (C \times 1.8) + 32$$

Convert Fahrenheit readings to Celsius by subtracting 32 from the Fahrenheit reading and dividing it by 1.8:

$$C = (F - 32)/1.8$$

| Celsius (Centigrade) | Fahrenheit |
| --- | --- |
| 36.0 | 96.8 |
| 36.5 | 97.7 |
| 37.0 | 98.6 (normal) |
| 37.5 | 99.5 |
| 38.0 | 100.4 |
| 38.5 | 101.3 |
| 39.0 | 102.2 |
| 39.5 | 103.1 |
| 40.0 | 104.0 |
| 40.5 | 104.9 |
| 41.0 | 105.8 |
| 41.5 | 106.7 |
| 42.0 | 107.6 |

From Perry AG, Potter PA, Ostendorf WR: *Nursing interventions & clinical skills*, ed 6, St Louis, 2016, Mosby.

## Volume Equivalents: Liquid Conversion

| | | |
|---|---|---|
| 30 mL | = | 1 oz (fl) = 2 tbsp (T) = 6 tsp (t) |
| 15 mL | = | ½ oz = 1 T = 3 t |
| 1000 mL | = | 1 quart (qt) = 1 liter (L) |
| 500 mL | = | 1 pint (pt) |
| 5 mL | = | 1 tsp (t) |

From Kee J, Hayes E, McCuistion L: *Pharmacology: a nursing process approach*, ed 8, Philadelphia, 2015, Saunders.

## ■ COMMON LABORATORY TEST VALUES

Critical abnormal test values must be reported to the physician as soon as they are received. Check your agency's list of what tests are considered critical.

### Complete Blood Count (CBC)

| | Conventional Units | SI Units |
|---|---|---|
| **Cell Counts** | | |
| ***Erythrocytes (red blood cells [RBCs])*** | | |
| Male adults | 4.5-6.0 T/L | $4.5\text{-}6.0 \times 10^{12}/L$ |
| Female adults | 3.7-5.2 T/L | $3.7\text{-}5.2 \times 10^{12}/L$ |
| Children (varies with age) | 3.9-5.2 T/L | $3.9\text{-}5.2 \times 10^{12}/L$ |
| ***Leukocytes (white blood cells [WBCs])*** | | |
| Total | $4\text{-}11 \times 10^3/\mu L$ | $4.0\text{-}11.0 \times 10^6/L$ |
| Differential | | |
| Myelocytes | 0% | 0/L |
| Band neutrophils | 0.0%-0.7% | $0.0\text{-}70 \times 10^6/L$ |
| Segmented neutrophils | 40%-73% | $1800\text{-}8000 \times 10^6/L$ |
| Lymphocytes | 20%-44% | $900\text{-}4800 \times 10^6/L$ |
| Monocytes | 3%-13% | $300\text{-}1400 \times 10^6/L$ |
| Eosinophils | 0%-6% | $0\text{-}660 \times 10^6/L$ |
| Basophils | 0%-3% | $15\text{-}50 \times 10^6/L$ |
| **Platelets** | | |
| | 140-400 B/L | $140\text{-}400 \times 10^9/L$ |
| **Reticulocytes** | | |
| | $24\text{-}84 \times 10^9/L$ (0.5-1.5% of erythrocytes) | $24\text{-}84 \times 10^9/L$ |
| **Hemoglobin** | | |
| Male adults | 14-17 g/dL | 8.7-10.6 mmol/L |
| Female adults | 12.5-15.0 g/dL | 7.6-9.3 mmol/L |
| Newborn | 9.4-20.5 g/dL | 5.8-2.7 mmol/L |
| Children (varies with age) | 10.3-16.0 g/dL | 6.4-9.9 mmol/L |
| Fetal total | Less than 2.0% of total | Less than 0.02% of total |
| **Hematocrit** | | |
| Male adults | 42%-52% | 0.42-0.52 |
| Female adults | 36%-46% | 0.36-0.46 |
| Newborn | 42%-65% | 0.42-0.65 |
| Children (varies with age) | 28%-44% | 0.28-0.44 |

Continued

Clinical Quick Reference

## Complete Blood Count (CBC)—cont'd

|  | Conventional Units | SI Units |
|---|---|---|
| **Corpuscular Values of Erythrocytes (for adults; values vary with age in children)** | | |
| MCH (mean corpuscular hemoglobin) | 26-34 pg/cell | 26-34 pg/cell |
| MCV (mean corpuscular volume) | 80-99 mm$^3$ | 80-99 fL/cell |
| MCHC (mean corpuscular hemoglobin concentration) | 32-37.5 g/dL | 320-375 g/L |

B/L, Billion per liter; T/L, trillion ($10^{12}$) per liter.
Adapted from Bope ET, Kellerman RD: *Conn's current therapy 2016*, Philadelphia, 2016, Saunders.

## Routine Urinalysis

| Component | Normal Value(s) |
|---|---|
| Color | Pale yellow to deep amber |
| Turbidity | Clear |
| Specific gravity | 1.005-1.030 |
| Osmolality | 275-295 mOsm/L |
| pH | 4.6-8.0 |
| Glucose | Negative |
| Ketones | Negative |
| Protein | Negative |
| Bilirubin | Negative |
| Red blood cells | None to 2 per high-power field |
| White blood cells | None to 4 per high-power field |
| Bacteria | None |
| Casts | Few or none |
| Crystals | None |

From Ignatavicius DD, Workman ML: *Medical-surgical nursing: patient-centered collaborative care*, ed 8, Philadelphia, 2016, Saunders.

## Laboratory Values for Chemistry Panel Test

|  | Conventional Units | SI Units |
|---|---|---|
| **Electrolytes** | | |
| Sodium, serum | 135-145 mEq/L | 135-145 mmol/L |
| Potassium, serum | 3.5-5.0 mEq/L | 3.5-5.0 mmol/L |
| Chloride, serum | 96-106 mEq/L | 90-106 mmol/L |
| Calcium, serum | 8.4-10.6 mg/dL | 2.10-2.65 mmol/L |
| **Chemical Values** | | |
| Glucose, serum (fasting) | 70-110 mg/dL | 3.9-6.1 mmol/L |
| Creatinine, serum | 0.6-1.2 mg/dL | 50-110 µmol/L |
| Uric acid, serum | 2.4-7.0 mg/dL | 143-416 µmol/L |
| Blood urea nitrogen (BUN), serum | 11-23 mg/dL | 8.0-16.4 µmol/L |
| Bilirubin, total serum | 0.3-1.1 mg/dL | 5.1-19 mmol/L |
| Carbon dioxide, serum | 24-31 mEq/L | 24-31 mmol/L |

## Laboratory Values for Chemistry Panel Test—cont'd

|  | Conventional Units | SI Units |
|---|---|---|
| Total protein, serum | 6.0-8.0 g/dL | 60-80 g/L |
| Albumin (A), serum | 3.5-5.2 g/dL | 35-52 g/L |
| Globulin (G), serum | 2.5 g% of protein | |
| A/G ratio | 1.5:1 to 2.5:1 | |
| Alanine aminotransferase (ALT), serum (SGPT) | 1-45 units/L | 1-45 units/L |
| Aspartate aminotransferase (AST), serum (SGOT) | 1-36 units/L | 1-36 units/L |
| **Cholesterol** | | |
| Total cholesterol, serum | <200 mg/dL | <5.20 mmol/L |
| Low-density lipoprotein (LDL) | 60-129 mg/dL | 600-1290 mg/L (LDL) cholesterol, serum |
| High-density lipoprotein (HDL) | >50-80 mg/dL | >500-800 mg/L (HDL) cholesterol, serum |
| Triglycerides, serum | 40-150 mg/dL | 0.4-1.5 g/L |

Pagana KD, Pagana TJ: *Mosby's manual of diagnostic and laboratory test reference*, ed 5, St Louis, 2014, Mosby.

## Normal and Abnormal Values for Arterial Blood Gases*

| Acid-Base Disturbances | pH | Paco$_2$ (mm Hg) | HCO$_3$ (mEq/L) | Pao$_2$ | Common Causes |
|---|---|---|---|---|---|
| None (normal values) | 7.35-7.45 | 35-45 | 22-26 | 80%-100% | |
| Respiratory acidosis | ↓ | ↑ | Normal | | Respiratory depression (drugs, central nervous system trauma), pulmonary disease (pneumonia, chronic obstructive pulmonary disease, respiratory underventilation) |
| Respiratory alkalosis | ↑ | ↓ | Normal | | Hyperventilation (emotions, pain, respirator overventilation) |
| Metabolic acidosis | ↓ | Normal | ↓ | | Diabetes, shock, renal failure, intestinal fistula |
| Metabolic alkalosis | ↑ | Normal | ↑ | | Sodium bicarbonate overdose, prolonged vomiting, nasogastric drainage |

*Values may vary slightly among laboratories.

From Pagana KD, Pagana TJ: *Mosby's manual of diagnostic and laboratory test reference*, ed 5, St Louis, 2014, Mosby.

## Reference Values for Therapeutic Drug Monitoring

| Therapeutic Test (Serum) for: | Range | Toxic Levels | Proprietary Test Name(s) |
|---|---|---|---|
| **Antibiotic Medications** | | | |
| Amikacin | 25-35 mg/mL | Peak > 35 mcg/mL*<br>Trough > 10-15 mcg/mL | Amikin |
| Gentamicin | 5-10 mg/mL | Peak > 10 mg/mL<br>Trough ≤ 4 mcg/mL | Garamycin |
| Tobramycin | 5-10 mg/mL | Peak > 10 mcg/mL<br>Trough ≤ 2-4 mcg/mL | Nebcin |
| Vancomycin | 5-35 mcg/mL | Peak 20-40 mcg/mL<br>Trough 5-10 mcg/mL | |
| **Anticonvulsant Medications** | | | |
| Carbamazepine | 4-12 mg/mL | >15 mg/mL | Tegretol |
| Ethosuximide | 40-100 mg/mL | >150 mg/mL | Zarontin |
| Phenobarbital | 15-40 mg/mL | 35-100 mg/mL (varies widely) | Luminal |
| Phenytoin | 10-20 mg/mL | >20 mg/mL | Dilantin |
| Primidone | 5-12 mg/mL | >15 mg/mL | Mysoline |
| Valproic acid | 50-100 mg/mL | >100 mg/mL | Depakene |
| **Analgesic Medications** | | | |
| Acetaminophen | 10-25 mcg/mL | >150 mcg/mL | Tylenol |
| Salicylate | 100-300 mg/mL | >300 mg/mL | |
| **Antineoplastic and Immunosuppressive Medications** | | | |
| Cyclosporine A | 100-400 ng/mL | >400 ng/mL | Sandimmune |
| Methotrexate (high-dose, 48 hr) | Variable | >0.5 mmol/L, 48 hr after dose | |
| Sirolimus (within 1 hr of 2-mg dose) | 5-15 ng/mL | Variable | Rapamune |
| Sirolimus (within 1 hr of 5-mg dose) | 10-28 ng/mL | Variable | Rapamune |
| Tacrolimus (FK-506), whole blood | 5-20 mg/L | >20 mg/L | Prograf |
| **Bronchodilators** | | | |
| Theophylline (aminophylline) | 10-20 mg/mL | >20 mg/mL | |
| **Cardiovascular Medications** | | | |
| Amiodarone (obtain specimen more than 8 hr after last dose) | 1-2 mg/mL | >2 mg/mL | Cordarone |
| Digoxin (specimen must be obtained 12 to 24 hr after last dose) | 0.8-2 ng/mL | >2.4 ng/mL | Lanoxin |
| Disopyramide | 2.8-7.5 mg/mL | >7 mg/mL | Norpace |
| Flecainide | 0.2-1 mg/mL | >1 mg/mL | Tambocor |
| Lidocaine | 2-6 mg/mL | >6 mg/mL | Xylocaine |
| Mexiletine | 0.5-2 mg/mL | >2 mg/mL | Mexitil |
| Procainamide | 4-8 mg/mL | >10 mg/mL | |
| Procainamide (measured as procainamide N-acetyl-procainamide) | 5-30 mg/mL | >30 mg/mL | |

## Reference Values for Therapeutic Drug Monitoring—cont'd

| Therapeutic Test (Serum) for: | Range | Toxic Levels | Proprietary Test Name(s) |
|---|---|---|---|
| Propranolol | 50-100 ng/mL | Not defined | Inderal |
| Quinidine | 2-5 mcg/mL | >6 mcg/mL | |
| Tocainide | 4-10 mcg/mL | Not defined | |

**Psychopharmacologic Medications**

| | | | |
|---|---|---|---|
| Amitriptyline | 100-250 ng/mL | >500 ng mL | Elavil |
| Bupropion | 25-100 ng/mL | >1200 ng/mL | Wellbutrin |
| Desipramine | 50-300 ng/mL | >400 ng/mL | Norpramin |
| Imipramine | 150-250 ng/mL | >500 ng/mL | Tofranil |
| Lithium carbonate (obtain specimen 12 hr after last dose) | 0.5-1.5 mmol/L | >1.5 mEq/L | Lithobid |
| Nortriptyline | 50-150 ng/mL | >500 ng/mL | Aventyl, Pamelor |

*A peak level may not be done.
Adapted from Bope ET, Kellerman RD: *Conn's current therapy 2016*, Philadelphia, 2016, Saunders.

## Therapeutic Monitoring of Anticoagulation Therapy

| | Normal | Therapeutic Range | Critical Level |
|---|---|---|---|
| Prothrombin time—may not be measured by the lab; if so, INR is used. | 11.0-12.5 seconds | 1.5-2 × normal | |
| International Normalized Ratio (INR) Used to monitor warfarin therapy | 0.8-1.1 | 2-3 | >5.5 |
| Activated partial prothrombin time (aPPT) Used to monitor heparin therapy | 30-40 seconds | 1.5-2.5 × normal | >70 seconds |

Clinical Quick Reference

## ■ MEDICATION ADMINISTRATION

### Relevant Abbreviations

| | | | | | | | |
|---|---|---|---|---|---|---|---|
| mL | = | milliliter | | PC, pc | = | after meals |
| fl oz | = | fluid ounce | | $\bar{c}$ | = | with |
| g, Gm, G, GM | = | gram | | $\bar{s}$ | = | without |
| gr | = | grain | | Bid, bid | = | twice a day |
| gtt | = | drop | | Tid, tid | = | three times a day |
| kg | = | kilogram | | Qid, qid | = | four times a day |
| µg, mcg | = | microgram | | q4h, q6h, q8h | = | every 4, 6, 8 hours |
| mEq | = | milliequivalent | | PRN | = | whenever necessary |
| mg | = | milligram | | NPO | = | nothing by mouth |
| l, L | = | liter | | STAT | = | immediately |
| $\overline{SS}$ | = | one-half | | IM | = | intramuscularly |
| T, tbsp | = | tablespoon | | IV | = | intravenously |
| t, tsp | = | teaspoon | | Subcut, SubQ | = | subcutaneously |
| <* | = | less than | | SL, subl | = | sublingual |
| >* | = | greater than | | IVPB | = | intravenous piggyback |
| PO, po, os | = | by mouth | | KVO | = | keep vein open |
| AC, ac | = | before meals | | | | |

*Use not recommended.

| TABLE **5.1** | The Joint Commission Minimum "Do Not Use" List of Abbreviations | |
|---|---|---|

| Do Not Use | Potential Problem | Use Instead |
|---|---|---|
| U (unit) | Mistaken for "0" (zero), "4" (four), or cc | Write "unit" |
| IU (international unit) | Mistaken for IV (intravenous) or the number 10 (ten) | Write "international unit" |
| Q.D., QD, q.d., qd (daily) | Mistaken for each other | Write "daily" |
| Q.O.D., QOD, q.o.d., qod (every other day) | Period after the Q mistaken for "I" and the "O" mistaken for "I" | Write "every other day" |
| Trailing zero (X.0 mg) [NOTE: Prohibited only for medication-related notations] Lack of leading zero (.X mg) | Decimal point is missed | Never write a zero by itself after a decimal point (X mg), and always use a zero before a decimal point (0.X mg) |
| MS | Can mean "morphine sulfate" or "magnesium sulfate" | Write "morphine sulfate" or "magnesium sulfate" |
| MSO$_4$ and MgSO$_4$ | Confused for one another | |

The Joint Commission, 2016. Reprinted with permission.

### The Joint Commission's Lists of Dangerous Abbreviations, Acronyms, and Symbols

A "minimum list" of dangerous abbreviations, acronyms, and symbols has been approved by The Joint Commission (TJC). The items in Table 5.1 must be included on each accredited organization's "Do Not Use" list.

The Institute for Safe Medication Practices (ISMP) has published a list of dangerous abbreviations (available at http://www.ismp.org) relating to medication use that it recommends should be explicitly prohibited. Two nurses usually must double-check the following before administration: heparin, insulin, parenteral chemotherapeutic agents, patient-controlled analgesia, and epidural pumps. Medications requiring a double check may vary by institution.

### Six Rights of Medication Administration

**Right medication.** Check the prescriber's order, and check the label with the medication administration record three times.

**Right dose.** Check the prescriber's order, check the dosage on the medication label three times, and calculate the correct amount to give as per the order.

**Right time.** Check the prescriber's order, and check the date and time on the medication administration record order three times. Check the expiration date of the medication.

**Right route.** Check the prescriber's order and verify the route of administration three times on the medication administration record.

**Right patient.** Check the armband name and number with the medication administration record sheet just before administering the drug, and ask the patient to state his or her name.

Each unit/dose/drug should be checked with the medication administration record, verifying each of the first four rights:
- As the medication is taken from the patient's drawer.
- As the medication is placed, still in its package, in a paper cup or on a small tray.
- Just before opening the package to administer the dose to the patient.

**Right documentation.** Document the drug **after** it has been given.

## Six Responsibilities for Medication Administration

1. Take a complete drug history.
2. Assess the patient for drug allergies.
3. Teach the patient about the drug and side effects to report.
4. Determine the reason the patient is receiving the drug.
5. Be aware of potential interaction with other drugs or foods.
6. Document effect of each drug you administer.

## Safety Guidelines to Prevent Medication Errors

When preparing to administer medications:
- Ask yourself why this drug is prescribed for this patient. Know the drug, the patient, and all of the patient's medical conditions.
- Before preparing medications, verify which patients are nothing by mouth (NPO) or off the unit.
- Verify that the medication orders on the medication administration record (MAR) have been checked against the prescriber's orders (if paper chart).
- If the patient is a child or an older adult, review the special precautions to be considered.
- Become familiar with the "high-alert drug list" from your facility's pharmacy. Be extra careful when administering a drug that is on this list. Be aware of look-alike and sound-alike drugs.
- Become familiar with the list of abbreviations that are no longer to be used, and ask for verification from the prescriber as to what is intended by the abbreviation if it appears in a written order.
- Plan ahead, and do not rush when preparing medications for administration.
- Prepare medications for administration in as distraction-free an environment as possible.
- Follow the Six Rights of medication administration every time you prepare and give medications.
- Check each medication with the order thoroughly three times before giving it to the patient.
- Ask before crushing a drug if you do not know whether it can be safely administered after crushing.
- If a crushed medication is prepared in the medication room, label the medication container with the medication, dose, date, and time. If an electronic health record (EHR) is in use, take the pill packaging to the room for bedside bar code scanning.
- Clarify with the prescriber any illegible writing in a drug order.
- Do not administer a drug if it is not clearly and correctly labeled with name and amount of the drug contained.
- Do not unwrap a unit-dose drug before you are at the patient's bedside and ready to administer the medication.

- Check any questionable order or unfamiliar drug or dosage with the pharmacist.
- If an ordered drug dosage seems odd, question it and check the order with the pharmacist or physician.
- Check pertinent laboratory values, and assess for side effects of the drug before giving the next dose.
- If a dosage calculation has to be made for a heart medication, insulin, heparin, or an anticancer drug, have the calculation repeated by another nurse and compare the results.
- Review the patient's MAR for any possible drug interactions.
- Know which medications require a double check and the signature of two nurses.
- Keep the drug in its original container. Discard leftover portions of unused medication from single-dose packages into designated containers.
- Become aware of drugs with similar names, and carefully check the original order.
- Question an excessive dosage increase in a patient's medication.
- Be familiar with every drug you administer. Look it up if you can't remember the information you need to administer it safely.
- Date multiple-dose medication vials as you open them.

At the time of medication administration to the patient:

- Use two patient identifiers. Verify the name, birth date, and/or number on the patient's armband with the information on the MAR each time you administer medications to the patient.
- Check the MAR and the chart for noted allergies, and question the patient before administering medications.
- Check each drug at the bedside with the patient's MAR before administering the medication. Electronic systems require bar code scanning of the patient's armband and each medication at the bedside.
- If the patient questions the drug or dose you are about to give, stop and check the situation.
- Sign that a medication has been given only after the patient has received it.
- Do not leave a medication dose at the patient's bedside.
- Document only after the patient has actually taken the medication.

When working with the patient for error prevention:

- Teach the patient about the drugs he or she is taking and the importance of proper identification of the medication before it is taken.
- Familiarize the patient with the color and shape of each medication, but consider that generic forms of the drug may differ. Instruct the patient to ask the pharmacist if a refill looks different from the last one.
- Obtain a complete drug history from the patient, including herbals, over-the-counter medications, and supplements.
  If a medication error occurs, always report it!

## Check Those Lab Tests!

When preparing to administer medications, you should know the laboratory test values relative to the action or potential adverse effects of each drug. For some drugs you will be checking to see if the medication is effective; for others, checking indicates if the drug is at a therapeutic level in the patient's body. Many drugs can affect kidney function, liver function, or bone marrow and blood cell function; laboratory tests are checked to verify whether adverse effects are occurring. Some medications will need alteration in dosing based on liver or kidney function. Checking your patient's lab values first thing during the shift will save you time later. Become familiar with the laboratory test values that should be checked when giving various medications and assessment data. Here is a list of common medications, or types of medications, appropriate assessments, and the test values to be checked. This is not a complete list. Check your drug handbook for other specific test values that should be checked for a particular medication.

| Medication | Laboratory Test Value to Check and Assessments |
| --- | --- |
| Digoxin (Lanoxin) | Serum digoxin, K+, apical pulse |
| Lasix | K+, urine output, BP |
| Procainamide | Serum level, ECG strip—Q-T interval |
| Heparin | aPTT |
| Warfarin (Coumadin) | INR, PT |
| Antibiotics | WBC count, liver function, renal function, culture and sensitivity report |
| Tobramycin | Serum peak and trough levels, renal function, hearing loss |
| Gentamicin | Liver functions—AST, ALT, bilirubin; renal function, hearing loss |
| Vancomycin | Kidney functions—BUN, creatinine; serum peak and trough levels |
| Amikacin | Therapeutic level; BUN, creatinine |
| Anticonvulsants | Specific drug serum level, CBC, AST, ALT, bilirubin, BUN, creatinine |
| Theophylline, aminophylline | Serum theophylline level (bronchodilators), lung sounds |
| Antihypertensives | CBC, electrolytes, BP |
| NSAIDs, acetaminophen, ibuprofen | CBC, liver functions—AST, ALT; kidney functions—BUN, creatinine |
| Hypoglycemics, insulins | Serum glucose, finger-stick glucose |
| Cortisone, corticosteroids | K+, CBC, serum glucose |
| Cholesterol-lowering statins | Cholesterol, HDL, LDL, triglycerides, AST, ALT, CPK |
| Iron preparations | CBC, Hgb, Hct |

*ALT, Alanine aminotransferase; aPPT, activated partial prothrombin time; AST, aspartate aminotransferase; BP, blood pressure; BUN, blood urea nitrogen; CBC, complete blood count; CPK, creatine phosphokinase; ECG, electrocardiogram; Hct, hematocrit; HDL, high-density lipoprotein; Hgb, hemoglobin B; INR, International Normalized Ratio; LDL, low-density lipoprotein; NSAIDs, nonsteroidal anti-inflammatory drugs; PT, prothrombin time; WBC, white blood cell.*

## Choosing the Correct Needle Size

The larger the number of the gauge, the smaller the needle.

| For | Use |
| --- | --- |
| **Intradermal Injections** | |
| Intradermal skin test | 27 gauge, ½ in |
| **Subcutaneous Injections** | |
| Allergy injection | 27 gauge, ½ in or ⅜ in |
| Immunization (some) | 25 gauge, ⅜ in |
| **Intramuscular Injections** | |
| Thin solutions | 23-25 gauge, 1 to 1½ in* |
| Antibiotic | 22 gauge, 1 to 1½ in* |
| Oil-based solution | 21 gauge, 1 to 1½ in* |

*Length depends on size of patient and the injection site chosen; larger patients need a longer needle to reach the proper depth.

## Sites for Intramuscular (IM) and Subcutaneous (Subcut) Injections

Avoid the dorsogluteal site whenever possible. The risk of hitting the sciatic nerve is great in this area and it is not a recommended site.

A  **Deltoid**

B  **Ventrogluteal**

C **Vastus Lateralis**

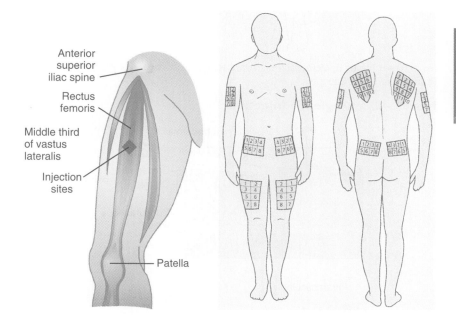

D **Rectus Femoris**    E Subcutaneous Rotation Sites

(From Kee J, Hayes E, McCuistion L: *Pharmacology: a nursing process approach*, ed 8, Philadelphia, 2015, Saunders.)

## Common Sites for Intradermal Injections

Forearm is most common.

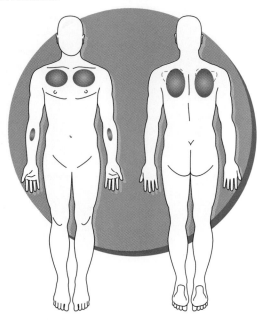

(From Kee J, Hayes E, McCuistion L: *Pharmacology: a nursing process approach*, ed 8, Philadelphia, 2015, Saunders.)

## Needle–Skin Angle for Injection

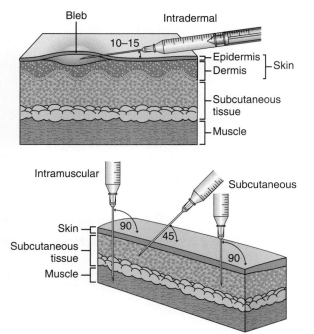

(From Kee J, Hayes E, McCuistion L: *Pharmacology: a nursing process approach*, ed 8, Philadelphia, 2015, Saunders.)

## Dosage and Solution Calculation Formulas

### BASIC DRUG CALCULATIONS FORMULA

$$\frac{D \quad \text{(desired)}}{H \quad \text{(on hand)}} \times V \quad \text{(vehicle, drug form)}$$

*Example:*

Order: amoxicillin 100 mg PO q6h
Available: amoxicillin 250 mg/5 mL

$$\frac{D}{H} \times = \frac{100 \text{ mg}}{250 \text{ mg}} \times 5 \text{ mL}$$

$$= \frac{500}{250} = 2 \text{ mL amoxicillin}$$

### RATIO AND PROPORTION

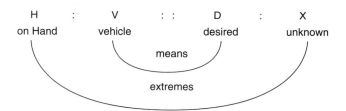

| H | : | V | : : | D | : | X |
|---|---|---|---|---|---|---|
| on Hand | | vehicle | | desired | | unknown |

means

extremes

*Example:*

Order: amoxicillin 100 mg PO q6h
Available: amoxicillin 250 mg/5 mL

$$
\begin{array}{ccccccc}
H & : & V & : : & D & : & X \\
250 \text{ mg} & : & 5 \text{ mL} & : : & 100 \text{ mg} & : & X \text{ mL}
\end{array}
$$
$$250 \text{ X} = 500$$
$$X = 2 \text{ mL amoxicillin}$$

### BODY WEIGHT (KILOGRAMS)

To change pounds to kilograms, divide by 2.2.
*Example:* Change 44 pounds to kg

$$44 \div 2.2 = 20 \text{ kg}$$
$$\text{Dosage/kg/day} = \text{dosage/day}$$
$$(\text{Dosage} \times \text{kg} = \text{dose/day})$$

*Example:*
Order: drug 6 mg/kg/day in four divided doses

$$6 \text{ mg} \times 20 \text{ kg} \times 1 \text{ day} = 120 \text{ mg/day}$$
$$120 \div 4 = 30 \text{ mg per dose}$$

From Kee J, Hayes E, McCuistion L: *Pharmacology: a nursing process approach*, ed 8, Philadelphia, 2015, Saunders.

## Major Drug Categories by Generic Name Endings

| Generic Name Ending | Example Generic Name(s) | Type of Drug | Common Action |
|---|---|---|---|
| -pril | lisinopril | Angiotensin-converting enzyme (ACE) inhibitor | Antihypertensive that relaxes arterial vessels |
| -sartan | losartan | Angiotensin receptor blocker | Antihypertensive that blocks action of vasoconstriction effects of angiotensin II |
| -olol, -alol, and -ilol | atenolol, labetalol, carvedilol | Beta blocker | Antihypertensive/antianginal that blocks beta-adrenergic receptors in vascular smooth muscle |
| -statin | atorvastatin | Antilipemic | Inhibits HMG-CoA reductase enzyme, thereby reducing cholesterol synthesis |
| -dipine | amlodipine | Calcium channel blocker | Antihypertensive/antianginal that produces relaxation of coronary smooth muscle and vascular smooth muscle; dilates coronary arteries |
| -afil | sildenafil | Phosphodiesterase type 5 inhibitor | Vasodilator that promotes a penile erection; relaxes pulmonary vessels, treating pulmonary hypertension |
| -floxacin | ciprofloxacin | Broad-spectrum anti-infective | Inhibits bacteria by interfering with DNA |
| -prazole | esomeprazole | Proton pump inhibitor | Suppresses gastric secretions, preventing gastric reflux and gastric and duodenal ulcers |
| -tidine | famotidine | Block histamine-2 ($H_2$) receptor | Inhibits histamine at $H_2$-receptor sites, decreasing gastric secretions |
| -azole | fluconazole | Antifungal | Causes direct damage to fungal membrane |
| -cyclovir | acyclovir | Antiherpetic | Interferes with DNA synthesis, causing decreased viral replication |
| -pam | diazepam | Antianxiolytic | Central nervous system depression |
| -micin | gentamicin | Aminoglycoside antibiotic | Bactericidal |
| -thromycin | azithromycin | Macrolide antibiotic | Bacteriostatic or bacteriocidal |
| -cillin | ampicillin | Penicillin antibiotic | Inhibits synthesis of cell wall |
| -cycline | doxycycline | Tetracycline antibiotic | Inhibits protein synthesis of bacteria |

## Major Drug Categories by Generic Name Endings—cont'd

| Generic Name Ending | Example Generic Name(s) | Type of Drug | Common Action |
|---|---|---|---|
| -arin | heparin, warfarin | Anticoagulant | Blocks conversion of thrombin and fibrinogen to fibrin |
| -azosin | terazosin | Antihypertensive | Inhibits sympathetic vasoconstriction |
| -cristine | vincristine | Antineoplastic | Causes metaphase arrest |
| -dopa | levodopa/ carbidopa | Antiparkinsonian agent | Replaces dopamine |
| -azine | chlorpromazine | Antipsychotic agent | Depresses cerebral cortex |
| -cyclovir | acyclovir | Antiviral agent | Interferes with viral DNA synthesis |
| -dronate | risedronate | Bone resorption inhibitor | Decreases rate of bone resorption |
| -tropium | tiotropium | Bronchodilator | Relaxes bronchial smooth muscle |
| -phylline | aminophylline | Respiratory smooth muscle relaxer | Produces bronchodilation; exact mechanism unknown |
| -oxin | digoxin | Cardiac glycoside | Increases cardiac output and force of contraction; decreases heart rate |
| -fate | sucralfate | Cytoprotective agent | Adheres to peptic ulcer site and absorbs pepsin |
| -sone | prednisone | Steroid | Decreases inflammation |

Adapted from a presentation by Barb Bancroft at the California Vocational Nurse Educators Conference in Sacramento, CA, April 25, 2008.

## High-Alert Medications

The following drugs can be dangerous if given in error. Be especially careful when administering these drugs. Be certain that there is a patient indication for the drug; that you are aware of the action, side effects, and adverse effects of the drug; and that you have assessed for those effects before giving the next dose. Check pertinent lab values before giving the drug. For cardiac drugs, check vital sign parameters to ensure safe administration.

- Amphotericin B, IV
- Antiepileptic drugs, injection, IV
- Antipsychotic drugs, injection
- Cardiac drugs, IV
- Chemotherapy agents
- Corticosteroid drugs, oral, injection, IV
- Dextrose, hypertonic solution IV
- Epinephrine, injection, IV
- Epoprostenol (Flolan), IV
- Heparin, low-molecular-weight heparin
- Insulin, subcutaneous, IV*
- Lasix, IV

- Lidocaine, IV
- Magnesium sulfate, injection
- Methotrexate, oral, use other than for oncology patients
- Narcotic drugs, oral, injection, IV
- Norepinephrine, IV
- Opium, tincture
- Oxytocin, IV
- Nitroprusside sodium, injection
- Oral hypoglycemic drugs
- Potassium chloride, injection
- Potassium phosphates, injection
- Promethazine, IV
- Sedative drugs, injection, IV
- Sodium chloride injection, greater than 0.9% concentration
- Sterile water for injection in vials larger than 100 mL
- Total parenteral nutrition solutions

*Insulin doses should always be checked with another nurse after the dose is drawn up and before it is administered.

## Insulins
## TYPES AND ACTIONS

| Preparation | Brand Name | Onset (hr) | Peak (hr) | Duration (hr) |
|---|---|---|---|---|
| **Rapid Acting** | | | | |
| Insulin aspart injection | NovoLog | 0.25 | 1-3 | 3-5 |
| Insulin lispro injection | Humalog | 0.25 | 0.5-1.5 | 5 |
| Insulin glulisine injection | Apidra | 0.3 | 0.5-1.5 | 3-4 |
| Insulin human inhalation powder | Afrezza | Immediate | 0.25 | 3 |
| **Short Acting** | | | | |
| Regular human insulin injection | Humulin R | 0.5 | 2-4 | 5-7 |
| | Novolin R, ReliOn R | 0.5 | 2.5-5 | 8 |
| **Intermediate Acting** | | | | |
| Human insulin isophane suspension NPH/ | Humulin N | 1.5 | 4-12 | 16-24+ |
| Insulin zinc suspension | Novulin N | 3-4 | 6-12 | 12-18 |
| (lente) | ReliOn N | 1.5 | 4-12 | 24 |
| **Long Acting (Also Called Basal Insulins)** | | | | |
| Insulin glargine injection | Lantus* | 2-4 | None | 24 |
| Insulin detemir injection | Levemir | 1 | 6-8 | 5.7-24 |

## TYPES AND ACTIONS—cont'd

| Preparation | Brand Name | Onset (hr) | Peak (hr) | Duration (hr) |
|---|---|---|---|---|
| **Combination Insulin** | | | | |
| 70% Insulin aspart prota-mine suspension/30% insulin aspart injection | NovoLog Mix 70/30 | 0.25 | 1-4 | 24 |
| 75% Insulin lispro prota-mine suspension/25% insulin lispro injection | Humalog Mix 75/25 | 0.25 | 1-4 | 24 |
| 70% Human insulin isophane suspension (NPH)/30% human insulin injection (regular) | Humulin 70/30, Novolin 70/30 | 0.5 | 2-12 | 24 |
| 50% Human insulin isophane suspension (NPH)/50% human insulin injection (regular) | Humulin 50/50 | 0.5 | 3-5 | 24 |
| **Basal Insulins/Concentrated Insulins** | | | | |
| Human insulin injection (concentrated U-500) | Humulin R U-500 | 0.5 | 4-8 | 13-24 |
| Insulin degludec injection (U-200) | Tresiba | 0.5-1.5 | 9 | 24-48 |
| Insulin glargine injection (U-300) | Toujeo | | | 30+ |

*Never mix Lantus with any other insulin.

Adapted from Ignatavicius DD, Workman ML: *Medical-surgical nursing: critical thinking for collaborative care*, ed 8, Philadelphia, 2016, Saunders; and Lamos EM, Younk LM, Davis SN: Concentrated insulins: the new basal insulins, *Therapeutics Clin Risk Management* 12:389–400, 2016.

## HYPOGLYCEMIA VERSUS HYPERGLYCEMIA

| | Hypoglycemia (<60 mg/dL) | Hyperglycemia (>250 mg/dL) |
|---|---|---|
| Cause | Too much insulin<br>Skipped or delayed meals<br>Too much exercise | Too little insulin<br>Overeating<br>Emotional stress<br>Illness, infection, stroke, heart attack, pregnancy |
| Early symptoms | Sweating, shaking, weakness<br>Headache, dizziness<br>Hunger | Excessive thirst<br>Frequent urination<br>Fatigue, weakness |
| Late symptoms | Numbness of lips or tongue<br>Difficulty concentrating<br>Irritability, mood changes<br>Blurred vision, pallor<br>If untreated: seizures, coma | Nausea, vomiting, abdominal pain<br>Flushed, dry skin<br>Fruity breath, drowsiness, lethargy<br>Loss of appetite, general aching<br>If untreated: labored breathing, coma, ketoacidosis |

Adapted from *Mosby's PDQ for LPN*, ed 43, St Louis, 2017, Mosby.

Clinical Quick Reference

## GUIDELINES FOR INSULIN ADMINISTRATION

- Check all insulin orders with the chart.
- Verify the patient's current blood glucose level per glucometer reading or lab work. Assess the patient for signs of hyperglycemia or hypoglycemia. Symptoms of **hyperglycemia** include nausea; vomiting; abdominal cramps; fatigue; increased thirst; increased urination; increased hunger followed by anorexia; weakness; dry mouth; acetone breath; and rapid, deep respirations. Signs of **hypoglycemia** include sweating; cold, clammy skin; feelings of numbness in fingers, in toes, and around mouth; rapid heartbeat; headache; nervousness; shakiness; faintness; slurred speech; hunger; vision changes; unsteady gait; weakness.
- Recheck blood sugar level by glucometer if above signs and symptoms are observed.
- Rapid-acting insulins should not be given until the patient's food tray has been delivered.
- Gently roll and invert the bottle to mix and ensure even drug particle distribution before withdrawing the solution from the vial.
- Check date on vial to be certain the insulin is in-date.
- When mixing regular and long-acting insulin, put air into the long-acting insulin vial and then put air into the regular insulin and draw up the correct amount of the regular insulin; draw up the exact amount of the long-acting insulin last.
- Always have another nurse verify the type and dosage of each insulin ordered as you prepare the injection.
- Use only an insulin syringe (insulin syringes are measured in units of insulin). Newer high-concentration insulins require the use of a 1-mL syringe (tuberculin syringe). Make sure to identify what concentration of insulin is being used.
- Inject at a 45- to 60-degree angle.
- Rotate injection sites to prevent lipodystrophy. Do not massage the site after injection. Use one site area daily for 1 week and then rotate to a new site. Keep a record of injection sites. Sites within an area should be 1½ inches apart. Abdominal sites are preferred for consistent absorption.
- If the patient gives his or her own insulin at home and is able to administer it in the hospital, allow the opportunity to do so.
- Never give any type but regular insulin by IV infusion.
- Watch for signs of hypoglycemia around the time that the insulin given is expected to peak (see the "Types and Actions" section under "Insulins" in this chapter). Give an oral carbohydrate snack if symptoms occur and blood glucose reading is low. Milk and crackers or 4 ounces of orange juice are commonly given. Do not give orange juice if the patient is a dialysis patient; orange juice has a high potassium content. If available, protein in the snack is best.
- Report hypoglycemic reactions to the staff nurse and your instructor immediately.
- Reassess blood glucose within 15 minutes.
- Continue to monitor the patient.
- Teach how to use an insulin pen if that is to be the mode of insulin delivery:
  - Screw on a new needle.
  - If pen requires priming to remove air, follow directions for priming.
  - Turn the dial knob on the end of the pen to the correct number of units.

- Insert the needle under the skin.
- Press the button on the end of the pen.
- Count to five before removing the needle from the skin.

### Digitalis Therapy

Digitalis is given to strengthen myocardial muscle action and slow the heart rate. Drug toxicity occurs frequently with this drug. **Early signs of toxicity** include anorexia, diarrhea, headache, confusion, fatigue, irritability, drowsiness, halos around lights, and green or yellow vision. **Further signs of toxicity** include cardiac arrhythmia (particularly bradycardia), depression, and convulsion. **A below-normal level of serum potassium predisposes the patient to digitalis toxicity.**

### NURSING CONSIDERATIONS

- Auscultate the apical pulse for 60 seconds to detect changes in rate or rhythm.
- If the heart rate is less than 60 or more than 100 beats/min, check the physician's orders for a notation as to whether the dose should be given or whether it should be withheld until the physician has been notified. Assess for other signs of toxicity before calling the physician (dose is held if toxicity is present).
- Check the last laboratory test level of digitalis and the last serum potassium level before administering the dose. Assess for signs of hypokalemia: muscle weakness, fatigue, anorexia, confusion, weak pulse, and nausea.
- Assess total medication regimen to determine possible interactions of digitalis with other drugs.
- If the patient is taking both digitalis and a diuretic that is not potassium sparing, potassium supplementation should be administered.

### PATIENT TEACHING

- Digitalis preparations should be taken at the same time each day.
- Check the pulse for a full minute before taking each dose.
- Report signs of digitalis toxicity; pay attention to early signs.
- Report any new irregular rhythm or abnormal pulse rate to the physician.
- Watch for signs of potassium depletion (hypokalemia). (Teach the signs.)
- Do not skip doses of the prescribed potassium supplement.
- If a digitalis dose is missed, do not take an extra dose without consulting the physician.
- Keep follow-up appointments with the physician.

### Steroid (Cortisone) Therapy

- Once-a-day steroid doses are given between 7:00 AM and 8:00 AM for best results, because this is when the body normally releases these hormones.
- Check for possible interactions with other drugs the patient is receiving.
- Insulin dosages may have to be adjusted when the patient is receiving steroids.
- Administer oral steroids with food or milk to minimize gastric irritation.
- Patients who are on nothing-by-mouth (NPO) status and are receiving parenteral steroids should be monitored for gastric bleeding. Medications to protect the gastric mucosa are usually given concurrently.
- Do not omit steroid dosages. If a dose has been inadvertently skipped, consult the physician.

- If the patient has been receiving steroids for 1 week or longer, the dosage must be tapered slowly rather than discontinued abruptly.
- Observe for infection, and protect the patient from exposure to infection while receiving steroids. Steroids can mask infection by suppression of the immune system.
- Assess for potassium imbalances and glucose imbalances.
- Increase calcium intake. Teach the patient receiving long-term steroid therapy measures to help prevent osteoporosis.
- Encourage regular eye examinations when the patient is receiving long-term therapy; steroids can cause cataracts and glaucoma.
- Assess for Cushing syndrome symptoms: moon face, buffalo hump, hirsutism, and edema.
- Observe for side effects of steroid therapy: nausea, abdominal pain, hypertension, pathologic fractures, osteoporosis, delayed wound healing, headache, mood changes, insomnia, and dizziness on standing.

## Anticoagulant Therapy

Your patient may receive heparin by continuous intravenous (IV) infusion, intermittent IV injection, or subcutaneous injection. Consider the following points:

- Protamine sulfate is the antidote for heparin overdose and should be kept on hand on the unit.
- The effectiveness of heparin therapy is judged by the extension of usual clotting time to 2.0 to 2.5 times normal (approximately 60 to 70 seconds). The activated partial thromboplastin time (aPTT) or partial thromboplastin time (PTT) is used to determine the clotting time. The result should be no more than 2.0 to 2.5 times the control time. The test should be done before therapy is begun and then repeated periodically, depending on how much heparin the patient is receiving. Lab monitoring of therapeutic levels is only done for IV infusions. **All heparin dosages should be checked with another nurse as they are prepared for IV injection.**
- Heparin subcutaneous injections are given in the abdominal fat at least 2 inches from the umbilicus in the area between the iliac crests.
- Enoxaparin (Lovenox) is a low-molecular-weight heparin for injection that is widely used. Blood tests are not required with this medication. Platelet levels are monitored with any form of heparin because of the risk of heparin-induced thrombocytopenia (HIT).
- Do not aspirate before injecting the heparin, because aspiration causes tissue trauma and bruising.
- Wait 10 to 15 seconds after injecting before removing the needle.
- Do not massage the area, because massaging causes increased bruising.
- Ice may be applied for 5 minutes to prevent bruising if this is a problem for the patient.
- Rotate the injection site from side to side.
- Be careful with IV starts, lab draws, and other activities that may cause bleeding or bruising. Frequent blood pressure monitoring can also cause bruising.
- Monitor the patient closely for signs of increased bleeding or hemorrhage, such as bloody urine (hematuria); dark, tarry stools (melena); bleeding of surgical wounds; bleeding gums; nosebleeds (epistaxis); hematomas; bloody sputum; bruising (ecchymosis); increased vaginal bleeding; neurologic changes; and signs and symptoms of hypovolemic shock.

- Patients who have been treated with heparin are often started on warfarin sodium (Coumadin) orally before the heparin is discontinued. This is done because it takes 3 days for the warfarin levels in the blood to build up to an effective anticoagulant level. Low-molecular-weight heparin may be given for use at home until therapeutic warfarin levels are achieved.
- Warfarin therapy's effectiveness is judged by the prothrombin time (PT) test. The result will be reported as an International Normalized Ratio (INR). Normal is 1.0. When recurrent systemic emboli are treated with warfarin, the INR is kept between 2.0 and 3.0. If used for prosthetic valve prophylaxis, the therapeutic levels are 3.0 to 4.0. The antidote for warfarin overdosage is injectable vitamin K.
- Rivaroxaban (Xarelto), apixaban (Eliquis), or dabigatran (Pradaxa) may be used instead of warfarin. These anticoagulant medications are not dosed by laboratory testing.
- Patients may also be started on antiplatelet aggregation medications such as clopidogrel (Plavix), aspirin, ticlopidine (Ticlid), dipyridamole (Persantine), prasugrel (Effient), or ticagrelor (Brilinta).

## PATIENT TEACHING
- Aspirin may be ordered with other antiplatelet or anticoagulant medications. Check with your physician before taking additional nonsteroidal anti-inflammatory drugs (NSAIDs) or salicylates.
- Avoid situations that could cause injury and bleeding, including contact sports. An electric razor may be used rather than a safety razor. Use a soft toothbrush, and avoid vigorous nose blowing.
- Many medications interact with warfarin; consult the physician regarding the possible interaction with other medications and supplements.
- Keep the amount of green vegetables containing vitamin K consistent in the diet.
- Limit alcohol intake.
- Take the medication at the same time each day.
- Inform all physicians and dentists that you are taking an anticoagulant.
- Wear an ID band stating that an anticoagulant is being taken.
- If bleeding occurs, apply pressure for 5 to 10 minutes and call the physician.
- Schedule follow-up tests to determine the effect of anticoagulant therapy.

# ■ INTRAVENOUS THERAPY

## Calculating Intravenous Flow Rates
### INTRAVENOUS FLOW RATE: CONTINUOUS—METHOD I
Amount of fluid ÷ hours to administer = mL/hr:

$$\frac{mL/hr \times gtts/mL \; (IVset)}{60min/hr} = gtts/min$$

*Example:*
Order: 1000 mL of 5% dextrose in ½-normal saline ($D_5$ ½NS) in 8 hr
IV set: macrodrip, 10 gtt/mL
1000 mL ÷ 8 hr = 125 mL/hr

$$\frac{125 \, mL/h \times \overset{1}{\cancel{10}} \, gtts/mL}{\underset{6}{\cancel{60}} \, min/hr} = 21 \, gtts/min$$

Clinical Quick Reference

## INTRAVENOUS FLOW RATE: INTERMITTENT—VOLUMETRIC PUMP

$$\text{Amount of solution} \div \frac{\text{Min to administer}}{60 \text{ min/hr}} = \text{mL/hr}$$

*Example:*
Order: 5 mL of drug solution in 100 mL of 5% dextrose in water ($D_5W$) in 45 min
Volumetric pump: 140 mL/hr to deliver 105 mL in 45 min

$$105 \text{ mL} \div \frac{45 \text{ min}}{60 \text{ min/hr}} \text{ (invert divisor and multiply)}$$

$$= 105 \times \frac{\overset{4}{\cancel{60}}}{\underset{3}{\cancel{45}}} = 140 \text{ mL/hr}$$

## INTRAVENOUS FLOW RATE: INTERMITTENT—SECONDARY SETS: BURETROL AND ADD-A-LINE

$$\frac{\text{Amount of solution} \times \text{gtts/mL (set)}}{\text{Min to administer}} = \text{gtts/min}$$

*Example:*
Order: 5 mL drug solution in 50 mL of $D_5W$ in 30 min
IV set: Buretrol (60 gtt/mL)

$$\frac{55 \text{ mL} \times \overset{2}{\cancel{60}} \text{ gtts}}{\underset{1}{\cancel{30}} \text{ min}} = 110 \text{ gtts/min}$$

## INTRAVENOUS FLOW RATE: CONTINUOUS—METHOD II

$$\frac{\text{Amount of fluid} \times \text{gtts/mL (IV set)}}{\text{H to administer} \times \text{min/h (60)}} = \text{gtts/min}$$

*Example:*
Order: 1000 mL of $D_5W$ in 10 hr
IV set: microdrip, 60 gtt/mL

$$\frac{\overset{100}{\cancel{1000}} \text{ mL} \times \overset{1}{\cancel{60}} \text{ gtts/mL}}{\underset{1}{\cancel{10}} \text{ h} \times \underset{1}{\cancel{60}} \text{ min/h}} = 100 \text{ gtts/min}$$

From Kee J, Hayes E, McCuistion L: *Pharmacology: a nursing process approach*, ed 8, Philadelphia, 2015, Saunders.

### Intravenous Flow Rate Chart

**Administration Sets Delivering 10 gtt/mL**

| Amount to be infused (mL) | 1000 | 1000 | 1000 | 1000 |
|---|---|---|---|---|
| Time of infusion (hours) | 12 | 10 | 8 | 6 |
| Rate of flow (gtt/min) | 14 | 17 | 21 | 28 |

## Intravenous Flow Rate Chart—cont'd

### Administration Sets Delivering 15 gtt/mL

| Amount to be infused (mL) | 1000 | 1000 | 1000 | 1000 |
|---|---|---|---|---|
| Time of infusion (hours) | 12 | 10 | 8 | 6 |
| Rate of flow (gtt/min) | 21 | 25 | 31 | 42 |

### Administration Sets Delivering 20 gtt/mL

| Amount to be infused (mL) | 1000 | 1000 | 1000 | 1000 |
|---|---|---|---|---|
| Time of infusion (hours) | 12 | 10 | 8 | 6 |
| Rate of flow (gtt/min) | 28 | 33 | 42 | 56 |

### Administration Sets Delivering 60 gtt/mL (Microdrip)

| Amount to be infused (mL) | 250 | 250 | 500 | 1000 |
|---|---|---|---|---|
| Time of infusion (hours) | 24 | 12 | 12 | 24 |
| Rate of flow (gtt/min) | 10 | 21 | 42 | 42 |

### Administration Sets Delivering 10 gtt/mL

| Amount to be infused (mL) | 50 | 50 | 50 |
|---|---|---|---|
| Time of infusion (minutes) | 20 | 30 | 60 |
| Rate of flow (gtt/min) | 25 | 17 | 8 |

### Administration Sets Delivering 15 gtt/mL

| Amount to be infused (mL) | 50 | 50 | 50 |
|---|---|---|---|
| Time of infusion (hours) | 20 | 30 | 60 |
| Rate of flow (gtt/min) | 38 | 25 | 12 |

### Administration Sets Delivering 20 gtt/mL

| Amount to be infused (mL) | 50 | 50 | 50 |
|---|---|---|---|
| Time of infusion (minutes) | 20 | 30 | 60 |
| Rate of flow (gtt/min) | 50 | 33 | 17 |

### Administration Sets Delivering 60 gtt/mL (Microdrip)

| Amount to be infused (mL) | 50 | 100 | 250 |
|---|---|---|---|
| Time of infusion (hours) | 2 | 8 | 6 |
| Rate of flow (gtt/min) | 25 | 12 | 42 |

## Calculation of Intravenous Intake

Start with the amount that was in the intravenous (IV) container at the beginning of the shift. If that entire amount infuses and a new container is hung, note the amount that is infused from the old container on the shift intake and output (I&O) sheet under "IV intake."

Next, at the end of the shift, note how much of the solution in the new container hung during the shift has infused. Draw a line and initial it with the time at that point on the container. Write the amount infused on the shift I&O sheet under "IV intake." Add the two amounts together to obtain the total IV intake for the shift.

To calculate the amount left to count in the IV container (for the next shift), subtract the amount infused from the new container from the total volume hung.

*Example:*

|  | Count | Infused |
|---|---|---|
| Count at beginning of shift | 450 mL | — |
| New solution added at 11:30 AM | 1000 mL | 450 mL |
| Amount infused at 2:00 PM | — | 325 mL |
| Amount left to count at end of shift | 675 mL | — |
| Total amount of IV intake | — | 775 mL |

**Intake from IV Pump**

|  |  |  |
|---|---|---|
| Rate × time in hours = mL intake | 100 mL/hr × 24 hr | 2400 mL |
| Volume of medication × # of doses = mL intake | 165 mL × 4 doses | 660 mL |
| Flush volume × # of flushes | 30 mL × 6 | 180 mL |
| *Total amount of IV intake* | — | *3240 mL* |

**"Smart" IV pumps will total the volume infused through the pump. Any infusions or line flushes not delivered via the pump will have to be added to the I&O total.**

## Intravenous Site Placement

- Identify suitable vein for placement of intravenous (IV) catheter. The cephalic, basilic, and median cubital veins are preferred in adults (Fig. 5.7).
- Use the most distal site in the nondominant arm, if possible. Choose a site that will least interfere with activities of daily living (ADLs).
- Clip arm hair with clippers and a sterile disposable head if site has considerable hair.
- Place extremity in dependent position if possible.
- Using a sterile IV start kit, place the tourniquet 4 to 6 inches above the chosen site. Do not apply tourniquet too tightly; check for radial pulse, indicating good blood flow distal to the tourniquet.

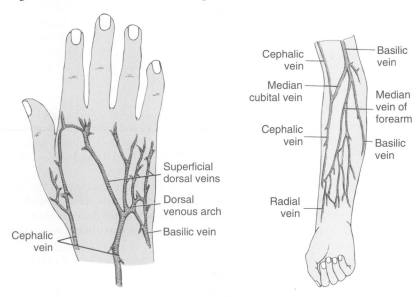

**FIG. 5.7** Veins for intravenous (IV) site placement. (From Perry AG, Potter PA, Ostendorf WR: *Nursing interventions and clinical skills*, ed 6, St Louis, 2016, Mosby.)

- Release tourniquet temporarily and prepare all equipment. Replace the tourniquet when ready to perform the puncture.
- Measures to increase venous distention include lightly tapping over the vein, stroking the extremity from distal to proximal below the proposed venipuncture site, having the patient open and close the fist and then leaving it closed, applying a moistened warm washcloth to the site for several minutes, and dangling the extremity for several minutes.
- Some facilities have vein visualization devices available to help locate veins.
- Follow correct procedure for cleansing the site and inserting the catheter, using standard precautions.

## Characteristics of Commonly Used Intravenous Fluids

| Solution | Tonicity | Calories | Use |
|---|---|---|---|
| 0.9% Normal saline (NS) | Isotonic | 0 | Fluid replacement, treatment of metabolic acidosis in presence of fluid loss, correction of sodium depletion; used before and after blood transfusion |
| 0.45% Normal saline (½NS) | Hypotonic | 0 | Electrolyte replacement of sodium and chloride |
| 5% Dextrose in water (D$_5$W) | Isotonic | 170 | Treatment of hypovolemia |
| 10% Dextrose in water (D$_{10}$W) | Hypertonic | 340 | Nutrient and electrolyte replacement |
| 5% Dextrose in 0.9% saline (D$_5$NS 0.9%) | Hypertonic | 170 | Treatment of circulatory insufficiency; fluid replacement |
| 5% Dextrose in 0.45% saline (D$_5$ ½NS) | Hypertonic | 170 | Maintenance of body fluids with nutrients and for treatment of fluid volume deficit |
| 10% Dextrose in 0.9% saline (D$_{10}$NS 0.9%) | Hypertonic | 340 | Nutrient and electrolyte replacement (sodium and chloride) |
| Hartmann solution | Isotonic | 0 | Extracellular fluid replacement for loss resulting from vomiting, diarrhea, or severe diuresis |
| 5% Dextrose in lactated Ringer solution (D$_5$RL) | Hypertonic | 170 | Electrolyte replacement plus nutrient |
| Lactated Ringer solution | Isotonic | 0 | Replaces sodium without increasing chloride levels |

## Setting up a "Piggyback" Minibag Medication

1. Check the medication order.
2. Verify that the medication is compatible with the main IV solution and its additives plus any other infusion connected to the IV line.
3. Remove the secondary (piggyback) tubing from its package, and close the roller clamp.
4. Label the tubing with the date.
5. Spike the piggyback medication container.
6. Squeeze the drip chamber and open the roller clamp to prime the tubing, keeping the connector sterile; close the roller clamp as soon as the tubing is primed. Any additional fluid loss results in a decrease in the amount of medication delivered.

7. Recheck the medication with the order or medication administration record (MAR).
8. Verify the patient identification. Perform the third check by bar code scanning the med or checking against the MAR.
9. Verify the patient's allergies and that there is no allergy to the piggyback medication.
10. Assess for side effects of a previous dose of the same medication. If adverse effects have occurred, withhold the medication and notify the physician.
11. Hang the piggyback minibag medication on the IV pole.
12. Lower the main IV container using the hanger that came with the secondary tubing set.
13. Cleanse the highest Y-site injection port below the drip chamber on the administration set tubing.
14. Attach the secondary tubing to the Y-site injection port.
15. Open the roller clamp on the secondary set, and regulate the flow to the desired rate.

**To set up the piggyback on the infusion pump: Remember that the setting on the infusion pump is in mL/hr.** Use the secondary screen (button for piggyback [PB] or "secondary") to program the proper flow rate. Enter the volume to be infused and the rate of infusion in mL/hr. Hang the piggyback higher than the primary bag of fluid. Follow the instructions for the brand of pump used in the facility. If in doubt, ask your staff nurse or your instructor to check the setting. Check the compatibility of the piggyback medication with all other fluids and meds flowing in the main line (patient-controlled analgesia [PCA] medication, primary bag medications, etc.). Consider whether the combined rate of flow is safe for the patient.

16. Chart the medication. Electronic health record (EHR) charting happens when the medication is scanned and the entry is verified.
17. Return when the time for the piggyback medication to infuse has ended.
18. Raise the primary IV container and re-regulate the flow to the ordered rate if not on a pump.
19. Note the amount of the piggyback medication that infused on the intake and output (I&O) sheet. Chart the time of the completion of infusion in the medical record.

## Intravenous Drug Compatibility

Anytime an intravenous (IV) drug is to be given by IV **push** injection into an existing IV line or by IV piggyback, compatibility with the solution that is infusing and any other drugs being infused must be checked before administration. Reasons for this caution are as follows:

- A physical incompatibility may occur. For example, when phenytoin (Dilantin) is injected into an IV line containing dextrose, a white precipitate forms, clogging the line and altering the chemistry of the medication.
- A chemical incompatibility may occur wherein one drug inactivates the other, making it ineffective. Or, the two drugs may combine into a harmful substance.
- Actions to be taken before IV drug administration, in addition to following the Six Rights and Responsibilities, include:
  1. Checking an IV compatibility chart or a drug handbook.
  2. Calling the pharmacist for information on compatibility.

3. Verifying that the solution used for dilution is compatible with the drug.
4. Flushing the IV line with a compatible solution before and after administering the drug.
5. **Administering the drug at the recommended rate for a bolus injection to prevent speed shock.**
6. Correctly flushing an intermittent IV cannula before and after administering a drug. The flush after administering the medication is injected at the same rate as the medication. During the flush, the medication that remains in the line is being administered.

## Intravenous Pumps: Tips for Use and Troubleshooting

- IV pumps vary greatly by manufacturer; obtain assistance as needed to learn the specific features.
- Check the medication, calculate the correct dosage, and determine the pump setting prior to entering the patient's room.
- For adult use, most pumps will deliver mL/hr. Set the pump for the correct rate in mL/hr.
- Pumps usually allow you to set a total volume; the machine's alarm will sound when it reaches that volume. (Use this feature to call you back at the end of the infusion or sooner as needed according to your clinical judgment.)
- Before you leave the room, check to ensure the following:
  - Patient is comfortable and there is no swelling or redness at the insertion site.
  - Appropriate clamps are open.
  - Intermittent dripping (not continuous) is observed in the drip chamber.
- Pumps can malfunction; assessment of site and equipment every 1 to 2 hours is a typical hospital policy.
- If the IV pump is continually alarming:
  - Check IV site for infiltration, clotting, etc.
  - Check tubing for kinks or air.
  - Check clamps and flow regulators.
  - Check IV bag to see whether there is fluid for infusion.
  - Make sure the pump is plugged into an electrical source.
  - Recheck settings on the pump.
  - Change the position of the patient's extremity (the IV may be positional).
  - Try turning the pump off and resetting it. Try another pump.

From Williams P: *Fundamental concepts and skills for nursing*, ed 5, St Louis, 2018, Saunders.

## Guidelines for Monitoring a Blood Transfusion

Students are not allowed to administer blood products but are often asked to monitor the patient who is receiving a blood transfusion. The student should accompany the nurse through each step of the process to become familiar with the procedure and the safeguards used when administering blood products.

## NURSING CONSIDERATIONS

- Double-check the physician's order.
- Verify that a consent form for blood administration has been signed.
- Assess to determine whether the patient has ever had a transfusion reaction.

- Administer any medications ordered to prevent transfusion reaction (e.g., antipyretic, antihistamine, or steroid).
- Verify that the correct size of IV cannula is in place. An 18-gauge cannula is preferable for trauma patients; a 20-gauge or 22-gauge cannula may be used for some blood products.
- Use a Y-type blood administration set of tubing with a filter. The blood container is attached to one side of the Y, and a container of normal saline is attached to the other side of the Y.
- **Before the container of blood is attached to the patient, the label is checked with the blood bracelet and ID band on the patient by two nurses.** Two identifiers are used, such as patient name, birth date, or hospital ID number. These identifiers verify that the correct patient, blood type, and unit match the patient's blood.
- The numbers must match among the blood container, the blood band on the patient's arm, and the information sheet accompanying the unit of blood from the blood bank. The ID check should include the following:
  - The patient's full name (check armband and ask the patient)
  - Patient's hospital number
  - Patient's birth date
  - Blood unit number
  - Blood group, Rh factor, and ABO designation
  - Expiration date
  - Type and crossmatch number
- Baseline vital signs, including temperature, are taken just before the blood transfusion is started.
- Use only saline (0.9% NaCl) before or during the transfusion in the same IV tubing. Start the saline slowly, before the blood arrives from the blood bank.
- Blood infusions must be started within 30 minutes of arrival on the unit; otherwise, return the blood to the blood bank. Blood may not be stored in the unit refrigerator.
- Stay with the patient for the first 15 minutes of the infusion. Monitor closely for signs of complications.
- Complications that may occur during infusion include high fever, sudden chills, headache, flushing, tachycardia, hypotension, itching, hives, rash, wheezing, shortness of breath, lower back pain, distention of neck veins, oppressive feeling in chest, and sense of impending doom. Should any of these symptoms occur, stop the infusion, do not allow any more blood to infuse, keep the IV patent by flushing the line or attaching another infusion, stay with the patient, and notify another nurse to call the physician. (The student also should notify the instructor.)
- Vital signs are taken after 15 minutes and then every half hour until the infusion is complete.
- **Do not allow blood to hang for more than 4 hours.**
- If a reaction occurs, follow the hospital protocol. For minor reactions, medications may be given and the unit continued. For major reactions, urine and blood samples may be needed and the unit of blood and tubing, must be returned to the blood bank with the appropriate information concerning the reaction.
- Monitor the patient closely for an additional hour after the transfusion, documenting vital signs. Continue to monitor during the following days for delayed reactions such as hematuria (blood in the urine).

## Principles for Administration of Total Parenteral Nutrition

- Placement of a central venous catheter must be verified by x-ray before the infusion of the total parenteral nutrition (TPN) solution is begun, unless the catheter was placed using fluoroscopy.
- Use an infusion pump to administer the TPN solution; start infusion slowly at first and then increase to the desired rate over a 24-hour period.
- Check the patient's tolerance of the infusion frequently during the first few hours.
- Monitor the patient's blood glucose every 4 to 6 hours per orders. Administer sliding-scale insulin as ordered for elevated blood glucose readings.
- Monitor continually for signs of complications, such as glucose intolerance, infection, fluid volume excess, phlebitis, and sepsis.
- Record the intake and output accurately.
- Never speed up the solution flow rate beyond that ordered, even if it falls behind for some reason.
- The TPN infusion must be tapered before being discontinued to prevent hypoglycemia.

## Principles for Administration of Peripheral Parenteral Nutrition (PPN) and Lipids

- Glucose concentrations 10% or less in IV nutrition solutions can be given in a peripheral vein.
- Additional carbohydrates are given to increase calorie intake via a lipid emulsion.
- The PPN and lipids usually run in separate primary IV lines and run through separate IV pumps. Lipids may require addition of a filter to the line.
- Make sure the IV site is clear and patent and the IV catheter is large enough to accommodate the volume of fluid to be infused, recognizing the lipids are thick. Usually a 20-gauge or larger catheter is sufficient.
- Start the infusions slowly according to facility protocol. Observe for possible allergic reaction. If symptoms occur, the allergy is usually to the lipids.
- Lipids may be infused with TPN also.
  Monitor the patient using the TPN guidelines listed above.

## ■ PERIOPERATIVE CARE

### Preparing the Preoperative Patient for Surgery

- Check that the surgical consent has been signed.
- Check whether a blood permit was required and, if so, that it was signed.
- Verify that the complete blood count, urinalysis, and other required diagnostic test data are available.
- Perform any bathing or skin prep needed. Have the patient put on a clean gown and have a surgical cap available.
- Check that the preoperative medications are available on the unit. Send the preoperative medication with the patient to the OR.
- Remove jewelry, and place all valuables in an envelope for safekeeping or give them to a family member. (A wedding band may be tied or taped in place.)
- Check and inquire about any piercings with body jewelry on any place on the body. If metal jewelry is left in place, the patient may be burned by the electrical cautery used during surgery. Remove the jewelry and secure it according to agency policy.

Clinical Quick Reference

- Remove all metal pins from hair.
- Complete the preoperative checklist, paper or electronic.
- One-half hour before the patient is expected to go to surgery, have him or her empty the bladder and remove dentures (if required).
- The area to be operated on (e.g., the right knee) is marked with indelible ink before the surgical procedure with the patient's verification, either in the patient's room or in the holding room in the surgical suite; follow agency protocol. This is best done before preoperative medication is administered.
- Prepare and administer any ordered preoperative medication at the time it is scheduled to be given, with the supervision of the instructor or nurse as required.
- Lower the bed, raise the side rails if sedation was given, place the call light within reach, and caution the patient not to get up.
- Finish charting in nurse's notes.
- When the transporter comes to take the patient to surgery, the patient is correlated with the transport slip, using two patient identifiers on the chart and patient ID band. Usually the name and birth date or hospital ID number are used. Correlate the procedure and site with the consent and the patient. The chart and the patient are correlated in the same manner.

## Safety Guidelines for Surgery

The Joint Commission has issued guidelines for preventing wrong site, wrong procedure, and wrong person surgery. The nurses on regular hospital units implement the following actions, which are part of a universal protocol.

### PREOPERATIVE VERIFICATION PROCESS

Verification of the correct person, procedure, and site should occur with the patient involved, awake, and aware, if possible:
- At the time of admission to the unit.
- Whenever care of the patient is transferred to another.
- Before the patient leaves the unit to enter the procedure or surgical suite.

### MARKING THE OPERATIVE SITE

A mark with a sufficiently permanent marker is placed at or near the incision site that will be visible after the patient's skin is prepared and draped. (Marking is exempted for single-organ surgery, cardiac catheterization, and tooth surgery, and on premature infants, on whom the marker may leave a permanent tattoo.) Preparation should not remove the mark. The marking is done by the person performing the procedure or surgery. Marking of the correct site should be performed before the patient leaves for the procedure room or surgical suite.

### DIAGNOSTIC TEST RESULTS ON HAND

Any x-rays, computed tomography (CT) scans, or magnetic resonance imaging (MRI) of the area to be involved in the procedure or surgery must be on hand in the procedure or surgical suite before the patient's arrival.

### "TIME-OUT" IMMEDIATELY BEFORE THE PROCEDURE IS STARTED

Before the procedure is begun, a "time-out" is called, wherein all members of the surgical or procedure team check the record, operative permit, and site marked; question the patient; and view any x-ray, CT, or MRI records to ascertain that the correct site is indeed marked. The procedure or surgery is not started until all questions or concerns are resolved. The unit nurse explains this protocol to the patient so that he or she will know what to expect. This process of procedural "time-out" is required for any invasive procedure regardless of where it is performed. A bedside insertion of a central line or chest tube requires a "time-out."

## Care and Assessment of the Postoperative Patient on Return to the Clinical Unit

- Obtain the report from the recovery room nurse who cared for the patient in the postanesthesia care unit (PACU).
- Note the time of return to the unit; quickly scan the post-operative orders.
- Transfer the patient to the bed and provide warmth.
- Take vital signs; compare them with previous data. Assess post procedure vital signs per agency protocol.
- Assess the wound and dressing; check drains; note amount and type of drainage; check or connect/compress wound suction devices.
- Position the patient for safety and comfort (usually on the side with the head up 15 to 30 degrees). Raise side rails per agency protocol until patient is fully alert.
- Assess color and temperature of the skin.
- Assess area/system involved in the procedure (e.g., check abdominal girth, distal pulses, movement of body parts).
- Check length of each tube for patency and function: urinary catheter, IV lines, chest tubes, and oxygen cannula. Attach tube to drainage device or suction as ordered.
- Check IV infusion for correct solution, additives, and rate of flow; assess site.
- Assess urinary status: time of last voiding, amount of fluids infused, bladder distention, urge to void, and amount of hourly output via catheter. **(Do not infuse IV fluid containing potassium until urine output is at least 30 mL/hr.)**
- Assess neurologic status: level of consciousness, orientation, ease of arousal, and ability to move extremities.
- Assess pain: verbal complaints, body language and time of previous analgesia, if any; medicate as needed per orders.
- Assess for nausea; medicate as needed per orders.
- Attach call light, and place emesis basin and tissues within reach.
- Assure the patient that the surgery is over and that he or she is safely back in the nursing unit.
- Allow family members to see the patient briefly.

## Guidelines for Traction, Pin, or Fixator Care

- Check the physician's order regarding the type of traction and amount of weight to be used.
- Assess the traction setup and verify that:
  - Weights are hanging free.
  - Patient's body is in correct alignment.
  - Traction components are positioned and functioning properly.
- **Assess for adequate circulation and sensation; check skin temperature.**
- Perform pin care as ordered if pins are in place.
- Do not use the fixator parts as leverage for moving the patient or a limb.

- Make the bed with an assistant from top to bottom, rather than side to side.
- Keep linens smooth under the patient.
- Obtain a trapeze bar so that the patient can assist with repositioning.
- Assess the area of injury for signs of infection; check for "hot" areas, drainage, and foul smell.
- Assess the need for pain medication on a regular schedule.
- Assess for systemic signs of infection (e.g., elevated white blood cell count, elevated temperature, increasing malaise).
- Offer bedpan frequently or on a set schedule per patient's elimination pattern.
- Track frequency of bowel movements, and take action if none occur for 3 days.
- Supervise range-of-motion exercises for other joints, especially in older patients.

### Postoperative Exercises to Prevent Complications

- Place the patient in a sitting position, preferably on the side of the bed so that lung expansion is not restricted by the mattress. Semi-Fowler or side position with the head of the bed elevated 30 to 40 degrees may be used.
- If the patient has a thoracic or an abdominal incision, splint the area with a small pillow or tightly folded towel; show the patient how to do this. Hold the splinting material tightly over the incision.
- Ask the patient to inhale as deeply as possible through the nose, hold the breath for a count of five, and then slowly exhale completely through the mouth; repeat four to six times.
- On the last deep breath, ask the patient to cough forcibly on exhalation. If he or she is unable to perform a full cough, ask the patient to exhale forcibly with the mouth open several times in a row to huff-cough and move secretions up the bronchial tree so that they can be expectorated.
- Repeat deep breathing and coughing at least every 2 hours, and ask the patient to deep breathe every hour, or whenever a commercial comes on the TV or a page of reading material is turned. To encourage the deep breathing, teach use of the incentive spirometer. **This is the most effective way to prevent postoperative respiratory complications.**

### USING THE INCENTIVE SPIROMETER CORRECTLY
Teach the patient to do the following:
- Place the mouthpiece in the mouth, and completely cover it with the lips.
- Take a slow, deep breath and hold it for at least 3 seconds.
- Remove the mouthpiece and exhale slowly, with the lips puckered.
- Breathe normally for a few breaths.
- Increase the inspired volume, if possible, by 100 mL with each breath.
- When maximal volume is attained, attempt to reach it 10 times, resting a few breaths in between each attempt.

### LEG EXERCISES
- Ask the patient to flex each foot firmly, pointing the toes toward the ceiling, and then to extend the foot fully and firmly. This action contracts and relaxes the calf and thigh muscles (gastrocnemius and quadriceps). Repeat five times.

- Ask the patient to rotate the ankles so that the toes draw circles, first in one direction and then the other. Repeat five times.
- Ask the patient to raise and lower the legs by bending and flexing at the knee; repeat five times. If the patient has an abdominal incision, raise the head of the bed 30 to 40 degrees before doing this exercise to relieve pressure on the abdominal muscles.
- Ask the patient to press the back of the knee against the mattress and then relax it if quadriceps-setting exercises are ordered. Repeat 10 to 12 times an hour.

These exercises should be used in addition to the sequential compression stockings.

## TURNING IN BED AND AMBULATION
- Assist the patient to turn in bed at least every 2 hours (preferably every hour) in a side-to-back-to-side pattern as permitted. Position the patient in proper body alignment, providing pillow support to the back, leg joints, and arms as needed.
- Prepare the patient by having him or her turn to the side and then push up to a sitting position, or raise the head of the bed with the patient supine and then pivot the legs and upper body so that he or she is sitting on the side of the bed.
- Allow the patient to sit on the side of the bed with the feet supported either on the floor or on a stool. (Place slippers or nonskid stockings on the feet.) Allow several minutes of sitting the first time up after surgery. Otherwise, a couple of minutes should be sufficient before the patient rises to a standing position.
- Assist the patient to a standing position, and allow time for stabilization of blood pressure before beginning ambulation. Support the patient appropriately.
- Assist with ambulation by providing the needed amount of support and assistance. Have the patient ambulate half the total distance planned because he or she will need to return to the bed or chair.
- Rubber-soled slippers are safest for ambulation. Provide warmth with a robe or other cover as needed. Remember to remove the robe before placing the patient back on the bed.

## Postoperative Hip Replacement Assessment
### BASIC ASSESSMENT
- Assess pain (e.g., related to surgery or chronic pain of degenerative joint disease).
- Assess blood drainage and wound site (e.g., drain at the surgical site with a suction device).
- Check position to prevent dislocation of the prosthesis (e.g., narrower end of abduction wedge is secured between the thighs if one is ordered; when seated, the hips are not flexed beyond a 90-degree angle). Newer surgical techniques may result in differences in positioning orders for hip surgery patients.
- Assess for signs of deep vein thrombosis (DVT) (e.g., Homans sign, pain, swelling).

## LAB VALUES TO CHECK
- Hematocrit and hemoglobin
- Electrolytes
- Prothrombin time, International Normalized Ratio (INR), or activated partial prothrombin time (aPPT)

## PATIENT PROBLEMS AND INTERVENTIONS
- Acute pain:
  - Assess for pain and encourage patient to report pain when it begins.
  - Reinforce instructions on patient-controlled analgesia (PCA).
  - Provide comfort measures: keep linens smooth and clean.
- Altered physical mobility:
  - Reposition every 2 hours or as needed.
  - Encourage range-of-motion (ROM) activity and exercises to improve muscle strength and joint flexibility.
  - Teach use of walker.
- Insufficient knowledge:
  - Explain that the patient should perform no flexion of the hip past 90 degrees, no internal rotation, and no adduction of the affected leg (or other ordered limitations).
  - Advise to report pain in hip, buttock, or thigh, or continued limp.

## ■ WHAT TO DO BEFORE YOU CALL THE PHYSICIAN

Be prepared with the information you need to tell the physician and use the SBAR (Situation, Background, Assessment, Recommendation) format. Incorporate the following information:
1. Who you are and where you are calling from
2. What happened:
   a. Relevant background information
   b. What you tried
   c. What you want
   d. If possible, prepare and organize other questions about less urgent matters to avoid another call:
      i. Take a full, current set of vital signs (e.g., several minutes before calling physician).
      ii. Obtain pulse oximeter reading and blood glucose value if patient has change of mental status.
      iii. Carefully assess patient so that you can fully describe the problem; have current lab results, vital signs, and the medication administration record (MAR) in hand.
      iv. Consult with charge nurse if you are unsure about urgency versus waiting (e.g., it's 3:00 AM; can this matter wait until the physician arrives for AM rounds?).
      v. Be prepared to report the baseline and any changes (e.g., usually alert and conversant, is now lethargic with slurred speech).
      vi. Seek an apparent cause for concern before calling (e.g., Foley catheter not draining because tube is kinked).
      vii. Try to resolve problem if possible (e.g., use position change or distraction for pain).

   viii.  Have pertinent lab values in front of you before you call.
    ix.  Have a blank sheet of paper available to jot notes and orders.

## ■ PERINATAL CARE

### Postpartum Assessment Guide

- Vital signs
- Breasts: engorgement, nipple condition, areas of warmth, redness, breastfeeding
- Uterus: fundus position, firmness
- Bowels: bowel sounds, bowel movement
- Bladder: distention, voiding
- Lochia: amount, color, clots, odor
- Episiotomy: appearance, edema, bruising, redness, drainage, approximation
- Perineum: presence of hemorrhoids—size, appearance
- C-section incision (if present): approximation, drainage, redness, tenderness
- Extremities: signs of thrombophlebitis, ability to ambulate
- Pain: location, character, severity, use of relief measures, need for analgesia
- Emotional status: family interaction, signs of depression
- Attachment: interest in newborn, eye contact, touch contact, ability to respond to infant cries

### Assisting the New Mother to Breastfeed

- Have the mother wash her hands before beginning.
- Position the mother comfortably sitting with her back and arm supported, supporting the infant with a cradle hold or football hold and pillows for proper height to breast **or** in a side-lying position with a pillow beneath her head, her arm above her head, and supporting the infant in side-lying position at breast level.
- Have her turn the infant's body to face her.
- Instruct her to stroke the infant's face with the nipple at the lower lip.
- Have her use a "C" position to hold the breast with the thumb above the nipple and the fingers below it; the nipple should not point upward.
- As the infant opens the mouth, have the mother insert the nipple and areola into the mouth.
- If breast tissue blocks the infant's nose, have the mother lift the infant slightly.
- Instruct the mother to nurse the infant for at least 10 minutes before changing to the other breast; if the infant is sucking vigorously, she should continue on this breast.
- Instruct the mother to break suction by placing a finger in the corner of the infant's mouth or indenting breast tissue at the mouth.
- Change position of the infant to nurse on the other breast.
- Have the mother place a safety pin on the strap for the opposite breast from where nursing began this session so she knows to start on the other breast next time.
- Instruct the mother to nurse at least every 2 to 3 hours initially. Exposing the nipples for 10 minutes to air and sunshine helps prevent or heal soreness.

### Estimation of Lochia Volume

**Scant:** Less than a 2-inch (5-cm) stain on perineal pad
**Light:** Less than a 4-inch (10-cm) stain on perineal pad
**Moderate:** Less than a 6-inch (15-cm) stain on perineal pad

**Large or heavy:** More than a 6-inch (15-cm) stain on perineal pad, or 1 pad saturated within 2 hours

**Excessive:** Saturation of a perineal pad within 15 minutes (report immediately)

From Leifer G: *Introduction to maternity & pediatric nursing*, ed 7, Philadelphia, 2015, Saunders.

## Fundus Massage

When the postpartum uterus is boggy or soft and is felt higher than the umbilicus, institute massage to encourage contraction. Check for bladder distention by palpation or bladder scan; if it is distended, have the mother void or catheterize her as needed before this procedure.

- With the woman in a supine position with the knees slightly flexed, lower the perineal pad so that you can observe the lochia as you massage the fundus.
- Place the outer edge of your nondominant hand just above the symphysis pubis and press downward slightly to anchor the lower portion of the uterus.
- Locate and massage the uterine fundus with the flat portion of the fingers of your dominant hand in a firm, circular motion.
- When the fundus is firm, keep the lower hand in place and gently push downward toward the vaginal outlet with the upper hand to expel blood and clots that have accumulated inside the uterus.
- Document the procedure and the result; note the amount of blood and clots expelled.

## Apgar Scoring

| Sign | 0 | 1 | 2 |
|---|---|---|---|
| Heart rate | Absent | Below 100 beats/min | 100 beats/min or higher |
| Respiratory effort | No spontaneous respirations | Slow; weak cry | Spontaneous, with a strong, lusty cry |
| Muscle tone | Limp | Minimal flexion of extremities; sluggish movement | Active spontaneous motion; flexed body posture |
| Reflex irritability | No response to suction or gentle slap on soles | Minimal response (grimace) to stimulation | Prompt response to suction and to gentle slap on sole of foot |
| Color | Blue or pale | Body pink, extremities blue | Completely pink (light skin) or absence of cyanosis (dark skin) |

A score of 8 to 10 requires just continued observation and support of adaptation; a score of 4 to 7 means the infant needs gentle stimulation such as rubbing the back; a score of 3 or lower means that the infant needs immediate active resuscitation.

Adapted from Leifer G: *Introduction to maternity & pediatric nursing*, ed 7, St Louis, 2015, Saunders.

## Umbilical Cord Care

The following procedure is to be done with each diaper change per facility protocol:

- Check clamp for tight closure.
- Assess for presence of three vessels unless dried.
- Lift the cord gently away from the abdomen for ease of cleaning all areas.
- Let the cord dry naturally, and keep it above the top of the diaper.
- Observe cord and abdominal attachment area for redness, discharge, or foul odor.
- Document observations and care.

# ■ GUIDELINES FOR ATTENDING CLINICAL IN A PSYCHIATRIC FACILITY

**Dress:** Street clothes, no lab coat or uniform. Avoid clothes with pictures or printing that could stimulate delusional thinking in the wrong direction by patients. Avoid tightly fitted clothes that are too revealing and sexually suggestive. Limit jewelry to stud earrings without dangles or hoops; no neck attire of any sort. Shoes must be low-heeled with closed toe area. Wear name pin for identification at all times. If forensic facilities are used, a color-coded dress code may be required.

**Grooming:** Hair should be pulled back and confined so that it cannot be grabbed easily.

**Safety:** Be alert to sudden sounds such as banging, loud voices, change of lighting, and new/strange smells. If these are encountered, turn toward that disturbance to assess the situation, and back up toward a safer area if need is indicated. Situational awareness is your best safety intervention.

## Symptoms of Post-traumatic Stress Disorder (PTSD)

PTSD can cause many symptoms, but watch for these:
* Reexperiencing symptoms
  * Flashbacks: reliving the trauma over and over, including physical symptoms
  * Bad dreams
  * Frightening thoughts
* Avoidance symptoms
  * Staying away from places, events, or objects that are reminders of the experience
  * Feeling emotionally numb
  * Feeling strong guilt, depression, or worry
  * Losing interest in activities that were enjoyable in the past
  * Having trouble remembering the dangerous event
* Hyperarousal symptoms
  * Being easily startled
  * Feeling tense or "on edge"
  * Having difficulty sleeping and/or having angry outbursts

From Post-Traumatic Stress Disorder (PTSD), http://www.nimh.nih.gov/health/publications/post-traumatic-stress-disorder-basics/index.shtml.

# ■ CARING FOR A PATIENT WITH ALZHEIMER'S OR OTHER DEMENTIA

* Allow extra time for accomplishing activities of daily living.
* Limit the number of choices you give.
* When the patient becomes agitated, use a distraction such as food, drink, music, or conversation.
* Match what you say with a corresponding action.
* Maintain eye contact and a comfortable posture.
* Identify what is triggering an undesirable behavior, and modify the environment.
* Label common items with pictures and/or words (e.g., toilet for bathroom door, lightbulb at the light switch, clothes on the closet door).

- Keep room well lit at all times without causing shadows.
- Involve patient in activities that require use of large muscle groups.
- Give the patient something to do or hold while you assist with carrying out a task (e.g., hold the toothpaste, an item of clothing, a washcloth).
- Approach the patient with a calm manner, smile, and gentle tone of voice.
- Use simple words and short sentences, and explain why you are there and what you are going to do. Use a picture flash card to help orient the patient to the task.
- Do not take combativeness or reluctance to do something personally; it is the disease causing the problem, not the patient.
- When the patient is resistant to doing something, try to figure out what he or she is feeling and express that to the patient. Sometimes this approach helps with cooperation.

# ■ NUTRITION

## Rehydration Formula for Dehydration from Vomiting and Diarrhea

Mix together:
2 quarts water
1 tsp. baking soda
1 tsp. salt
7 T. sugar
A packet of sugar-free Kool-Aid or other sugar-free drink mix may be added. Can be frozen into ice cubes or into ice pops.

## Alternative Seasoning Mix (Makes ⅓ Cup)

| | |
|---|---|
| 1 T. dry mustard | 5 tsp. onion powder |
| 1 tsp. thyme | 1 T. garlic powder |
| ½ tsp. white pepper | 1 T. paprika |
| ½ tsp. celery seed | |

Mix together. Store in a closed container.

## A Guide to Daily Food Choices

Use MyPlate (Fig. 5.8) from the U.S. Department of Agriculture (USDA) to help people eat better every day. General recommendations from the USDA (2015) for the general population include the following:
- Enjoying food but eating less of it
- Avoiding oversized portions
- Increasing intake of whole fruits, vegetables, and whole grains
- Choosing low-fat or fat-free dairy products
- Reducing intake of sodium
- Drinking water instead of sugary beverages
- Making physical activity an everyday occurrence
- Additional tips and resources, including recipes and interactive tools, are available at choosemyplate.gov.

Note the specific Dietary Guidelines from the USDA:

- **Fruits and vegetables:** Consume 2 cups of fruit and 2½ cups of vegetables daily. Make fruits and vegetables half of what is eaten at each meal. Choose fiber-rich fruits and vegetables.
- **Whole grains:** Consume 6 ounces daily. Eat three 1-ounce portions of whole grains. Choose whole, unsweetened grains when possible.
- **Dairy products:** Drink 3 cups of skim or low-fat milk, or eat the equivalent dairy products (e.g., low-fat yogurt, low-fat cheese).
- **Protein:** Eat 5½ ounces of poultry, lean meat, fish, beans, or nuts. Eat meat rarely. Choose lean meats and poultry. Bake, broil, or grill meat, poultry, and fish choices.
- **Oils and sweets:** Consume 6 teaspoons per day, used sparingly. Use healthful oils such as olive, canola, and safflower. Sugar should be limited. Keep total fat intake between 20% and 35% of calories, with most fats coming from sources of polyunsaturated and monounsaturated fatty acids, such as fish, nuts, and vegetable oils. Consume less than 7% of calories from saturated fatty acids and less than 300 mg/day of cholesterol, and keep *trans*–fatty acid consumption as low as possible.
- Calorie control is to be considered as well for a healthy diet. Combine a healthy diet with sufficient exercise to maintain a healthy weight.

### Choice Equivalents Within Each Food Group

Servings based on a 2000-calorie diet:

- **Fruits:** 2 cups of fruit a day. Eat a variety and use fresh, frozen, canned, or dried fruit rather than fruit juice. A serving could be 1 small banana, 1 medium orange, or ¼ cup of dried apricots or peaches.
- **Vegetables:** 2½ cups a day. In particular, select from all five vegetable sub-groups (dark green, orange, legumes, starchy vegetables, and other vegetables) several times a week. Eat portions of vegetables for lunch and dinner.

FIG. 5.8    MyPlate. (From U.S. Department of Health and Human Services/U.S. Department of Agriculture, 2016. www.choosemyplate.gov.)

- **Grains:** 6 ounces per day; 3-ounce equivalents a day of whole-grain products. Half the grains should be whole grains. One ounce is 1 slice of bread, 1 cup of breakfast cereal, or ½ cup of cooked rice or pasta.
- **Protein:** 5½ ounces of poultry, lean meat, fish, beans, or nuts per day. Equivalent servings of 1 ounce of meat, fish, or poultry are as follows: 1 egg, ¼ cup cooked beans, 1 tablespoon peanut butter, ½ ounce of nuts or seeds, and ¼ cup tofu. A 4-ounce serving of meat, fish, or poultry for dinner should be about the size of a normal deck of cards or the palm of the hand. Eat two 4-ounce servings of fish per week. Choose a variety of protein foods.
- **Dairy products:** 3 cups of milk per day; 1 cup of milk equals 8 ounces. Equivalent servings to 1 cup of milk are 1 cup of low-fat or nonfat yogurt; ½ ounce of low-fat cheese, such as Swiss, Gouda, Roquefort, and white string cheese; or 2 ounces of low-fat or fat-free processed cheese, such as American or Laughing Cow.
- **Fats:** 6 teaspoons per day. One teaspoon of liquid oil is equal to 1 teaspoon of tub margarine, 1 tablespoon of mayonnaise, or 2 teaspoons of light salad dressing.

## Key Recommendations

### ALL POPULATIONS

- Engage in regular physical activity, and reduce sedentary activities to promote health, psychological well-being, and a healthy body weight.
- Balance body weight in a healthy range; balance calories from foods and beverages with calories expended. Eat a more plant-based diet.
- Those who choose to drink alcoholic beverages should do so sensibly and in moderation—defined as the consumption of up to one drink per day for women and up to two drinks per day for men.
- Consume less than 1 g of sodium (approximately 1 tsp of salt) per day. Choose and prepare foods with little salt. At the same time, consume potassium-rich foods, such as fruits and vegetables. Age 51 and older: limit sodium to 1500 mg per day.

### CHILDREN AND ADOLESCENTS

Children 2 to 8 years of age should consume 2 cups per day of fat-free or low-fat milk or equivalent milk products. Children 9 years of age and older should consume 3 cups per day of fat-free or low-fat milk or equivalent milk products.

### WOMEN OF CHILDBEARING AGE WHO MAY BECOME PREGNANT

Eat iron-rich plant foods or iron-fortified foods along with vitamin C–rich foods. Consume adequate folate foods daily or adequate synthetic folic acid from a supplement.

### WOMEN IN THE FIRST TRIMESTER OF PREGNANCY

Consume adequate synthetic folic acid daily from fortified foods or supplements in addition to folate food forms.

### PEOPLE OLDER THAN 50 YEARS OF AGE

- Consume vitamin $B_{12}$ in its crystalline form (i.e., fortified foods or supplements).
- Older adults, people with dark skin, and people exposed to insufficient ultraviolet sunlight: consume extra vitamin D from vitamin D–fortified foods and/or supplements.

## Body Mass Index

The body mass index (BMI) is based on the relationship of weight to height. It is independent of body frame size. BMI is used to determine whether a person has excess fat. Body mass is calculated with the following formula:

$$BMI = \frac{Weight\ (lb)}{Height(in)^2} \times 705$$

In the adult, a score of 20 to 25 is within normal and is associated with the least risk of early death.

*Example:* A woman 5 feet 4 inches tall, weighing 122 pounds:

$$Height\ squared = 64in \times 64in = 4096$$
$$122 \div 4096 = 0.0297085$$
$$0.029785 \times 705 = 20.9$$

This woman's body mass index is 20.9.

## Therapeutic Diets

In the hospital setting, many types of diets are needed to address the needs of patients as part of the treatment plan. Renal diets, carbohydrate-consistent diets, National Dysphagia Diets (NDDs), and neutropenic diets are some of the diets offered. Below are some of the most common.

### CLEAR LIQUID DIET

**Purpose.** Provides an oral source of calories and electrolytes as a means of preventing dehydration and reducing colonic residue to a minimum.

**Indications.** The immediate postoperative period, acute debilitation, acute gastroenteritis, upper gastrointestinal lesions; also to reduce the amount of residue in the colon in preparation for bowel surgery barium enema, or after colon surgery.

| Type of Food | Foods Included | Foods Excluded |
|---|---|---|
| Beverage | Carbonated beverages, tea, coffee, strained fruit juice (apple, cranberry, cran-apple, grape, punch, powdered fruit beverage mixes, electrolyte replacement drinks) | Milk, milk drinks |
| Soup | Fat-free bouillon or broth, consommé | Any other |
| Dessert | Plain gelatin, Popsicles, fruit ice | Any other |
| Condiments | Sugar, honey, plain hard candy | Any other, caffeine, artificial sweetener |

### FULL LIQUID DIET

**Indications.** Oral surgery, mandibular fracture, plastic surgery to the face, esophageal strictures; also for acutely ill patients for whom chewing may be difficult, or other postoperative states in transition between a clear liquid and another diet; three to six small feedings a day are recommended.

**Contraindications.** Nausea, vomiting, distention, or diarrhea when advanced to this diet postoperatively; lactose intolerance.

| Type of Food | Foods Included | Foods Excluded |
|---|---|---|
| Beverage | Carbonated beverages, coffee, tea, fruit juices, milk, milk drinks, vegetable juices (strained), eggnog | None |
| Bread | None | All |
| Cereal | Soft-cooked cereals (gruels) | Any other |
| Fat | Butter, cream, margarine | Any other |
| Vegetables | Tomato juice, vegetable puree in soup | Any other |
| Meat, egg, cheese | Raw pasteurized eggs*; soft-cooked egg sometimes allowed | Any other |
| Soup | Broth, strained cream soups, yogurt | Any other |
| Dessert | Yogurt, custard, ice cream (plain), pudding, tapioca, sherbets, plain gelatin | Any other |
| Condiments | Pepper, salt, cinnamon, nutmeg, sugar, honey, hard candy, syrup, pureed meat and vegetables for soup only | Any other |

*Raw unpasteurized eggs should not be used because of the danger of *Salmonella* infection. In addition, the avidin in the egg white prevents the absorption of biotin.

Adapted from Peckenpaugh N, Poleman C: *Nutrition essentials and diet therapy*, ed 11, Philadelphia, 2010, Saunders.

## SOFT, LOW-FIBER (BLAND) DIET

**Indications.** Gastrointestinal disturbances, general physical weakness, or poor chewing ability.

**Note.** Soft diet contains whole pieces of food that are not chopped or pureed. Some elements of this soft diet may have to be adjusted in consistency to fit the needs of a particular patient (e.g., pureed meats, fruits).

| Type of Food | Foods Included | Foods Excluded |
|---|---|---|
| Beverage | Carbonated beverages, decaffeinated coffee or tea, milk, milk drinks | Alcoholic, cocoa, or caffeinated beverages |
| Bread | White or fine rye bread or rolls, soda crackers, waffles, graham crackers, muffins, cornbread | Whole-grain products, any breads with nuts, seeds, or dried fruits |
| Cereal | Cream of wheat or rice cereals | Whole-grain cereals, bran, cereals cooked with nuts, seeds, or fruits, hard or firm dry cereal |
| Fats | Butter, cream, margarine, salad dressing, gravy, mayonnaise, sour cream | Fried foods |
| Fruit | Fruit juices, ripe avocado, banana, cooked or canned apples, apricots, cherries, pears; all of the listed fruit without skin or seeds; dried fruit puree | Raw fruits, skins, or seeds; citrus juice or fruit; pineapple; cranberries |
| Vegetables | Cooked, pureed vegetables; vegetable juice | Raw vegetables or skins, broccoli, cabbage, cauliflower, mild or hot peppers, sauerkraut, avocado, tomatoes or tomato products |

| Type of Food | Foods Included | Foods Excluded |
|---|---|---|
| Potato or substitute | Potatoes, sweet potatoes, rice, spaghetti, grits, macaroni, noodles | None |
| Meat, eggs, cheese | Ground or tender nonstringy meat, fish, or chicken; eggs; cottage cheese; cheddar or American cheese; yogurt; tofu; and smooth peanut butter | Fried meat, chicken, or fish; strong cheeses; dried cooked beans; processed spicy meats |
| Soup | Puree from food allowed, all cream and broth soups | Whole vegetable or meat soups unless adjusted in consistency for patient, tomato-based soup, chili |
| Dessert | Custard, gelatin, angel food cake, tapioca, puddings, ice cream, cake, plain cookies, hard candy | Rich desserts, nuts, raisins, coconut |
| Condiments | Salt, white pepper, sugar, vinegar, sauces, gravy, ketchup, honey, syrup, jelly | Olives, pickles, popcorn, relishes, black pepper, strong spices, chili |

Data from Medline Plus: *Bland diet*. Updated December 2, 2011. http://www.nlm.nih.gov/medlineplus/ency/patientinstructions/000068.htm.

## American Heart Association Guidelines for a Heart-Healthy Diet and Lifestyle

The American Heart Association's recommendations include the following points:
- Consume an overall healthy diet.
- Maintain a healthy body weight by balancing calories consumed with calories burned.
- Be aware of your daily caloric requirements and increase awareness of the calorie content of various food portions.
- Obtain at least 30 minutes of physical activity each day. Do not smoke.
- Eat a variety of fruits and vegetables (not fruit juices), adding deeply colored ones such as spinach, carrots, peaches, and berries.
- Limit carbohydrate choices to whole-grain, high-fiber foods, decreasing refined grains such as white bread and white rice.
- Consume food-based sources of fiber (legumes, whole grains, fruits, and vegetables).
- No more than half of discretionary calories should come from added sugars.
- Have two servings of fish relatively high in omega-3 fatty acids twice a week. (Pregnant women and children should avoid mercury-contaminated fish.)
- Choose extra-lean meats and low-fat (<5 g total fat) or fat-free dairy products; limit intake of saturated fat, *trans*-fat, and cholesterol.
- Use non–animal-based sources of protein such as legumes and beans.
- Consume less than 10% of calories from saturated fats. Keep *trans*-fat consumption to no more than 3 g per day (based on a 2000-calorie diet).
- Take in few beverages and foods with added sugars, including high-fructose corn syrup.

- Keep sodium consumption down to 2300 mg daily; prepare foods with little or no salt. Middle-age and older adults, African-Americans, and those with hypertension should limit sodium intake to 1500 mg of sodium per day.
- Limit alcohol to one drink per day for women and two drinks per day for men (1 drink = 12 oz of beer, 4 oz of wine, 1.5 oz of 80-proof distilled spirits, or 1 oz of 100-proof distilled spirits).
- Take in vitamins A, C, D, E, and $B_{12}$ through vitamin-rich foods and/or supplements.
- At all times be aware of portion size; when eating out, select vegetables and fruits, and avoid foods prepared with added saturated or *trans*-fat, salt, and sugar.

Data from American Heart Association: Diet and lifestyle recommendations. Updated January 20, 2016. http://www.heart.org/HEARTORG/GettingHealthy/NutritionCenter/HealthyEating/The-American-Heart-Associations-Diet-and-Lifestyle-Recommendations_UCM_305855_Article.jsp.

## Low-Fat Diet

| Frequently Consumed High-Fat Foods | Alternative Foods |
|---|---|
| Fried foods | Roast, bake, grill, stir-fry, or broil foods when possible. Baste meats with broth or stock. Use nonstick cookware and an aerosol cooking spray. |
| Fatty meats (bacon, sausage, choice grade meats, poultry, frankfurters, luncheon meats) | Choose two or three servings of meat and shellfish or fish, with a daily total of about 6 oz. Choose a vegetarian entrée (dried beans, peas) at least once a week. Trim visible fat from meat; remove skin from poultry before eating. Choose beef grade "select," which contains less fat marbling; leaner cuts of meat include beef flank, sirloin, or tenderloin; loin pork chops. Marinate lean cuts of meat in lemon juice, flavored vinegars, or fruit juices. |
| Cheese (aged and cream cheeses) | Choose cheese with 6 g or less of fat per ounce, such as farmer's cheese. |
| High-fat snacks (chips, some crackers, dips) | Substitute with pretzels, low-fat crackers, air-popped popcorn. |
| Salad dressing, mayonnaise, sour cream | Use fat-free or reduced-fat salad dressings and sour cream. Substitute plain low-fat yogurt for mayonnaise or sour cream. Rely on mustard and salad greens to add moisture to sandwiches rather than high-fat spreads. |

| Frequently Consumed High-Fat Foods | Alternative Foods |
|---|---|
| Gravies | Use the paste method for making gravy or sauces (add flour or cornstarch to cold liquids slowly and blend well). |
| Homogenized whole milk products | Use skim milk, buttermilk, low-fat yogurt, and cottage cheese. |
| Margarine and seasonings such as lard, bacon, and ham | Use jam, jelly, or marmalade spread instead of butter or margarine. Season with herbs, lemon juice, or stock rather than lard, bacon, or ham. |
| Breads and cereals | Plain bread, rolls, graham crackers, matzoh, saltines, pretzels, most cereals. |

## DASH (Dietary Approaches to Stop Hypertension) Eating Plan

Research has shown that the DASH combination eating plan lowers blood pressure and therefore may help prevent and control high blood pressure. This diet is rich in fruits, vegetables, and low-fat dairy foods, and low in saturated and total fat. It is also low in cholesterol; high in dietary fiber, potassium, calcium, and magnesium; and moderately high in protein. The following DASH eating plan is based on 2000 calories a day. Depending on caloric needs, the number of daily servings in a food group may vary from those listed.

| Food Group | Daily Servings | Serving Sizes | Examples and Notes | Significance of Each Food Group to the DASH Diet Pattern |
|---|---|---|---|---|
| Grains, grain products | 7-8 | 1 slice bread ½ cup dry cereal ½ cup cooked rice, pasta, cereal | Whole wheat bread, English muffin, pita bread, bagel, cereals, grits, oatmeal | Major sources of energy, fiber |
| Vegetables | 4-5 | 1 cup raw leafy vegetables ½ cup cooked vegetable 6 oz vegetable juice | Tomatoes, potatoes, carrots, peas, squash, broccoli, turnip greens, collards, kale, spinach, artichokes, sweet potatoes, beans | Rich sources of potassium, magnesium, fiber |
| Fruits | 4-5 | 6 oz fruit juice 1 medium fruit ½ cup dried fruit ½ cup fresh, frozen, or canned fruit | Apricots, bananas, dates, oranges, orange juice, grapefruit, grapefruit juice, mangos, melons, peaches, pineapples, prunes, raisins, strawberries, tangerines | Important sources of potassium, magnesium, fiber |

| Food Group | Daily Servings | Serving Sizes | Examples and Notes | Significance of Each Food Group to the DASH Diet Pattern |
|---|---|---|---|---|
| Low-fat, non-fat dairy foods | 2-3 | 8 oz milk<br>1 cup yogurt<br>1.5 oz cheese | Skim or 1% milk, skim or low-fat buttermilk, nonfat or low-fat yogurt, part-skim mozzarella cheese, nonfat juice | Major sources of calcium, protein |
| Meats, poultry, fish | 2 or less | 3 oz cooked meats, poultry, fish | Select only lean; trim away visible fats; broil, roast, or boil, instead of frying; remove skin from poultry | Rich sources of protein, magnesium |
| Nuts, seeds, legumes | 4-5 per week | 1.5 oz or ⅓ cup nuts<br>½ oz or 2 tbsp seeds<br>½ cup cooked legumes | Almonds, filberts, mixed nuts, peanuts, walnuts, sunflower seeds, kidney beans, lentils | Rich sources of energy, magnesium, potassium, protein, fiber |

National Heart Lung and Blood Institute: What is the DASH eating plan? Available at http://www.nhlbi.nih.gov/files/docs/public/heart/new_dash.pdf.

## Sodium-Restricted Diet

Along with foods, the sodium content of medications and local water should be considered. Potent oral diuretics have lessened the need for severe limitation of sodium in the diet.

### INDICATIONS

Chronic heart failure, hypertension, atherosclerosis, edema, cirrhosis of the liver, or chronic kidney disease.

| Type of Diet | Sodium Per Day Allowed | Foods Excluded |
|---|---|---|
| No added salt | 4-5 g | No salty or high-sodium processed foods; do not add salt to food at the table; use only small amounts in cooking |
| Mild sodium restriction | 2-3 g | No added salt; no pickles, olives, bacon; restrict ham, chips, canned soups, salted nuts, smoked meats or fish, bouillon, frozen entrées, luncheon meats, processed cheese, regular peanut butter, instant cocoa or hot cereals, cooking wine, seasoning salts, soy sauce, Worcestershire sauce, meat extracts |

| Type of Diet | Sodium Per Day Allowed | Foods Excluded |
|---|---|---|
| Moderate sodium restriction | 1 g | Same foods restricted as in mild sodium diet; only low-sodium products are to be used; no restriction on commercially baked products; no cheese or canned or frozen vegetables containing salt; no more than 2 cups of milk |
| Severe sodium restriction | 500 mg | Same foods are restricted as in moderate sodium diet; only restriction is salt-free bread; no high-sodium fruits or vegetables such as celery, carrots, beets, artichokes, Swiss chard, greens, kale, spinach, white turnips, sauerkraut, hominy |

## High-Fiber Diet

Fiber increases fecal bulk, holds water, and binds calcium, magnesium, and other needed nutrients. The inclusion of high-fiber foods in the diet is recommended for patients on a general diet and for those with constipation. In addition, a high-fiber diet may be helpful in the treatment of diverticular disease. High-fiber foods include whole-grain breads and cereals, bran, oatmeal, wheat germ, millet, brown rice, cornmeal, legumes (dried beans), nuts, seeds, and fresh fruits, as well as vegetables with skins (e.g., apples, grapes, apricots, raw cauliflower, carrots, celery, cabbage, lettuce). Bananas, prunes, dates, figs, and rhubarb are good laxatives and high in fiber.

## High-Calorie, High-Protein, High-Vitamin Diet

This diet is indicated for underweight or malnourished patients. The normal diet is supplemented with foods high in protein, vitamins, and calories. Small, frequent feedings are best (six to eight per day). The caloric value can be 25% to 50% above normal (up to 3000 calories/day), and the protein increased to 90 to 100 g/day for adults who do not have renal insufficiency.

Cheeses, sauces, cream soups, potatoes, ice cream, pudding, and milk shakes may be used liberally. Prepared nutritional supplements such as Ensure, Ensure Plus, Sustacal, Boost, or Carnation Instant Breakfast may be used at meals or between meals. Supplementary vitamins may be indicated.

| Group | Number of Servings |
|---|---|
| Milk | 4 or more |
| Meat or meat substitutes | 3 or 4 |
| Breads and cereals | 4 to 8 |
| Fruits and vegetables | 4 or more |

## Gluten-Free Diet

Patients with celiac disease or sprue must completely avoid gluten. Those with gluten sensitivity should avoid gluten as much as possible. A gluten-free diet should not be used to promote weight loss. Some prescription drugs, vitamins, and over-the-counter drugs contain gluten. Patients should be told to consult their pharmacist.

Clinical Quick Reference

## FOODS ALLOWED

**Fruits and vegetables:** Fresh, frozen, and canned fruits and vegetables and their juices

**Meats and protein alternatives:** Fresh meat, fish, and poultry; eggs; dried beans and peas; nuts and seeds; tofu. Fresh turkey without additives.

**Milk products:** Milk, cream, buttermilk, yogurt, plain cheese, cream cheese, cottage cheese

**Grains:** Breads and baked goods made from gluten-free products, pastas made from rice, beans, corn, potato, quinoa, millet, soy, wild rice, and other gluten-free grains

**Cereals:** Puffed corn, amaranth, buckwheat, millet, rice, rice flakes or soy, hominy grits, soy grits, cream of buckwheat, cream of rice, puffed amaranth

**Rice:** Brown, white, basmati, jasmine, or wild rice; rice tortillas

**Corn:** Tortillas

**Fats and oils:** Butter, margarine, vegetable oils, lard, shortening, cream

**Desserts:** Gluten-free cakes, cookies, pastries; many ice creams, sorbets, sherbets, Popsicles, whipped toppings, egg custards, gelatin, most hard candies, most chocolate bars

**Beverages:** Cocoa drinks, soft drinks, juices, non-dairy soy; rice-, potato-, and nut-based beverages; teas, coffee; distilled alcoholic beverages such as rum, gin, whiskey, vodka, wines, and pure liqueurs; gluten-free beer, ale, and lager

**Sweet condiments:** Honey, jams, jellies, marmalade, molasses, corn syrup, maple syrup, sugar (white, brown, and confectioner's)

**Snack foods:** Plain popcorn, potato chips, corn chips, nuts, soy nuts, rice cakes, corn cakes, rice crackers

**Condiments:** Salad dressings without gluten-based ingredients, plain pickles, relish, olives, ketchup, mustard, tomato paste, pure herbs and spices, gluten-free soy sauce, vinegars (all but malt vinegar)

**Common baking ingredients:** Pure cocoa, baking chocolate, chocolate chips, carob chips and powder, cream of tartar, baking soda, yeast, brewer's yeast, vanilla

**Soups, sauces, and gravies:** Homemade broths, gluten-free bouillon cubes, cream soups and stocks made from allowed ingredients, sauces and gravies made from allowed ingredients

## FOODS TO AVOID

Barley

Rye

Oats (unless totally gluten free)

Couscous

Hydrolyzed protein

Wheat-based soy sauce

Meat extenders and vegetarian meal substitutes

Deli meats, hot dogs, sausages, imitation seafood products unless all natural

Marinades and sauces

Baked beans

Seasoned nuts

Flavored tofu

Malted milk

Cheese sauces, cheese spreads, flavored cheeses

Seasoned or flavored rice mixes, rice pilaf

Icing or frosting

Ice creams containing wheat or wheat-containing ingredients
Dried fruits
Candy bars and soft candies; licorice
Flavored teas, coffees, and herbal teas containing barley or barley malt
Undistilled alcoholic beverages, coolers
Some brands of potato chips
Seasoned popcorn
Pretzels and crackers (regular)
Soy and teriyaki sauce
Packaged dry salad dressing mixes
Many commercial salad dressings
Instant mashed potatoes
Worcestershire sauce
Malt vinegar
Hot cocoa mix
Seasoning mixes
Prefrozen French fries (dusted with flour)
Commercially produced soups and broths (contain wheat flour or hydrolyzed
    wheat protein)

---

*Data from Case S: *Gluten-free diet: a comprehensive resource guide*, Regina, Saskatchewan, Canada, 2008, Case Nutritional Consulting Inc.

## Lactose-Free Diet: Foods to Avoid

**Beverages:** Milk, ice cream, sour cream, yogurt,* soft cheeses, mayonnaise, cream cheese, half-and-half, whipped cream, cottage cheese, evaporated milk, condensed milk, dry milk powder, breakfast drinks

**Bread and pasta:** Bread, biscuits, pancakes, French toast, waffles, toaster pastries, doughnuts, sweet rolls, crackers, and cakes often contain lactose from milk products

**Sauces and toppings:** Salad dressings containing milk or whey, cheese sauces, butter, dips, whipped toppings, sauces containing milk or milk products

**Vegetables:** Any au gratin, scalloped, or creamed vegetables, and vegetables with cheese sauce

**Sweets:** Ice cream cake, frozen yogurt, milk chocolate, puddings, custards, sherbets and desserts with sweetened condensed milk; butterscotch, caramel, and toffee-flavored sweets, and some artificial sweeteners (check label)

**Other food products:** Many protein powders and bars, instant potatoes, soups, nondairy liquid and powdered coffee creamers, nondairy whipped toppings, some salad dressings, candies

---

*Yogurt with active live cultures decreases the lactose content of the product and may be tolerated.

## Principles for Administering Enteral (Tube) Feedings

- Always check for proper tube placement before beginning a feeding. If a nasogastric tube is newly placed, a chest x-ray is required to verify placement.
- Elevate the head of the bed 30 to 45 degrees, and leave it up for 30 to 60 minutes after the feeding. Keep the head of the bed elevated at all times if the feeding is continuous.

- Check for gastric residual before starting the next feeding or every 4 hours. Follow facility protocol regarding actions to take based on the amount of residual.
- If nausea occurs, stop the feeding and notify the physician.
- If persistent diarrhea occurs, notify the physician.
- Monitor bowel movements.
- Check skin turgor to be certain patient is not becoming dehydrated. Water in addition to the tube feeding may be ordered.
- Be alert to signs of hyperglycemia during the first few days of tube feeding.
- Flush the tubing with 30 to 50 mL of water, depending on fluid requirements, after each feeding and at least once per shift.
- When giving medications, flush the tubing with 10 to 30 mL of water initially and with 10 mL of water after each medication. Do not mix medications together.
- Use elixirs rather than crushed pills whenever possible. If pills have to be crushed, crush ahead of time and mix with warm water. Never crush a sustained-release medication.
- If tubing is clogged, check with a nurse for unit protocol on unclogging tubing. Using warm water and milking the tubing is sometimes sufficient; carbonated cola is used in some facilities, and cranberry juice is used in others.

## Giving Medication via Nasogastric or Small-Bore Tube*
### EQUIPMENT
- Clean gloves
- 50-mL barrel syringe
- Container for tap water
- pH test strip
- Stethoscope

### STEPS
- Check medication with medication administration record (MAR); verify patient name, allergies.
- Perform the Six Rights of medication administration.
- Prepare medication (i.e., use liquid form if possible; tablets must be finely crushed and diluted in water; timed-release capsule beads should not be crushed; the beads may appear very small but will easily clog tubing; consult with instructor or staff before administering).
- Assess presence of bowel sounds, abdominal distention, nausea, or vomiting.
- Elevate head of bed (HOB) 30 to 90 degrees.
- Verify tube placement (e.g., with a 50-mL syringe, gently aspirate a few drops of stomach contents and test with pH paper). For small-bore tube, check x-ray result for correct placement and that the tube is still inserted correctly by noting where the black line is in relation to the nostril per the initial note after insertion.
- Clamp tube to prevent excess air from entering tube.
- Draw up 30 to 50 mL of water*; unclamp tube and gently flush.
- Clamp tube; detach syringe and remove plunger; reattach barrel to use as funnel.
- Add liquid medication slowly and allow to instill; add water for flushing before the syringe is entirely empty to prevent excessive air from entering tube.

- Clamp tube for 30 to 60 minutes before reattaching to wall suction.
- Assess patient for nausea, fullness, and discomfort.
- Leave HOB elevated during procedure and for 30 to 60 minutes afterward.
- Clean and rinse syringe and water container; store at bedside.
- Document procedure and outcomes.

---

*Enteral practice recommendations published in the *Journal of Enteral and Parenteral Nutrition* state that sterile or purified water is recommended for medication administration. https://www.ismp.org/tools/articles/ASPEN.pdf

# ONLINE RESOURCES

*Note:* These listings are provided as aids for studying, class work preparation, and patient teaching. Be aware that websites come and go, and what follows are examples of online resources available for selected topics at the time of printing. The author and publisher do not endorse the websites listed.

## ■ RESOURCES FOR NURSING STUDENTS

### ARTERIAL BLOOD GAS TUTORIAL
http://www.ausmed.com.au/blog/entry/interpreting-abgs-simple-and-easy

### ASSERTIVENESS SKILLS
http://www.skillsyouneed.com/ps/assertiveness.html
http://www.ndsu.edu/counseling/self_help/assertiveness_skills/

### AUSCULTATION ASSISTANT
http://www.wilkes.med.ucla.edu/intro.html

### BEST PRACTICE GUIDELINES
https://www.guideline.gov/
http://rnao.ca/bpg/guidelines
http://rnao.ca/bpg

### CARDIAC INFORMATION
www.mendedhearts.org
www.blaufuss.org/
www.med.umich.edu/lrc/psb/heartsounds/
www.easyauscultation.com/heart-sounds

### CARE PLANS AND TEMPLATES
http://www.careplans.com/pages/lib/default.aspx?cid=6
http://www.rncentral.com/nursing-library/careplans
http://web.nmsu.edu/~ebosman/nursing/careplan.shtml

### CAREGIVER INFORMATION
www.caregiver.com
http://www.caregiversupportnetwork.com/
http://helpguide.org/home-pages/caregiving.htm

### COMPLEMENTARY AND ALTERNATIVE MEDICINE
http://www.mayoclinic.org/healthy-living/consumer-health/in-depth/alternative
    -medicine/art-20045267
http://nccam.nih.gov

## CONCEPT MAPPING
http://ojni.org/6_2/602/strategies.htm
http://www.ehow.com/how_5526833_make-nursing-concept-map.html
http://www.slideshare.net/nytenurse/concept-mapping-100669

## CULTURAL INFORMATION
http://babelfish.com (for translation)
http://depts.washington.edu/pfes/CultureClues.htm
https://ccnm.thinkculturalhealth.hhs.gov/
http://www.ccah-alliance.org/icetoolkit.html

## DETERMINING YOUR LEARNING STYLE
http://www.ldpride.net/learning-style-test.html
http://www.educationplanner.org/students/self-assessments/learning-styles-quiz
    .shtml

## DISABILITIES
www.aucd.org/
www.exceptionalnurse.com
www.washington.edu/doit/Careers/print.html?ID=314

## DISTANCE LEARNING AND DEGREE PROGRAMS
http://www.allnursingschools.com/nursing-careers/article/online-nursing-school/
http://www.accreditedschoolsonline.org/nursing-schools/online-degree-programs/
http://www.nursingdegrees.com/
www.rncentral.com

## DRUG CALCULATION HELP
www.dosagehelp.com
http://www.nursesaregreat.com/drug-calculations.php
www.testandcalc.com/quiz/index.asp

## ECG INFORMATION
http://cal.vet.upenn.edu/projects/lgcardiac/ecg_tutorial/introduction.htm
www.gwc.maricopa.edu/class/bio202/cyberheart/ekgqzr.htm
http://library.med.utah.edu/kw/ecg

## EVIDENCE-BASED NURSING
www.ahrq.gov/clinic/cpgsix.htm
www.guideline.gov
http://hsl.mcmaster.ca/resources/topic/eb/nurse.html
http://www.cochrane.org/what-is-cochrane-evidence
http://libguides.ohsu.edu/ebptoolkit
http://www.nursingcenter.com/evidencebasedpracticenetwork/home/tools
    -resources/collections/understandingevidencebasedpractice.aspx

## FLASHCARD PROGRAMS
http://www.cram.com/tag/nursing
http://quizlet.com/
http://www.studystack.com/Nursing

## FORUMS AND NETWORKING
http://onlinelpntorn.org/2011/40-best-forums-for-nursing-students/
http://allnurses.com/nursing-student
http://www.nursetogether.com/

## GENERAL MEDICAL INFORMATION
http://emedicine.medscape.com/
www.healthcentral.com
http://health.nih.gov
http://www.mayoclinic.org/patient-care-and-health-information
http://ods.od.nih.gov/Health_Information/How_To_Evaluate_Health
    _Information_on_the_Internet_Questions_and_Answers.aspx
www.medscape.com
www.nlm.nih.gov/medlineplus

## GENERAL NURSING RESOURCES
www.healthfinder.gov
http://www.practicalnursing.org/

## GENERAL REFERENCES
www.bartleby.com
http://www.medicinenet.com/medterms-medical-dictionary/article.htm
www.merriam-webster.com
http://medical-dictionary.thefreedictionary.com/

## GRANTS AND SCHOLARSHIPS
www.collegescholarships.org/grants/nursing.htm
http://edu.fastweb.com/v/o_registration/flow/step1?ref=google_nursing-1f
www.oshpd.ca.gov/HPEF
www.hrsa.gov/loanscholarships/scholarships/Nursing
http://minoritynurse.com/scholarships/

## NATIONAL COUNCIL LICENSURE EXAMINATION (NCLEX) INFORMATION AND STUDY TIPS
www.nclexinfo.com
www.ncsbn.org/nclex.htm
www.ncsbn.org/1268.htm
http://www.kaptest.com/NCLEX/Home/decision-tree.html
http://www.atitesting.com/Solutions/PostGraduation/nclex.aspx

## NUTRITIONAL INFORMATION
www.eatright.org
www.choosemyplate.gov

## PHARMACOLOGY HELP
http://www.nova.edu/optometry/pharmacy
http://nursingpharmacology.info/
http://web.utah.edu/umed/courses/year2/pharm/study/

### RESUME AND INTERVIEW TIPS
http://www.resume-now.com/lp/rnarsmnurs.aspx?cobrand=RSMN&tag=1209211
85946583&hitlogid=118244876&ref=9095&utm_source=PPCg&utm
_medium=SEMK&utm_term=how+to+write+a+nursing+resume&utm
_campaign=e-Nursing

### STRESS MANAGEMENT
http://helpguide.org/mental/stress_management_relief_coping.htm
http://holistic-online.com/Stress/stress_home.htm

### STUDY AIDS
http://www.studygs.net
http://www.studystack.com/Nursing
http://www.howtostudy.org/resources_subject.php?id=31

### VIDEOS
http://www.learnerstv.com/Free-Nursing-Video-lectures-ltv184-Page1.htm
http://www.nursingworld.org/FunctionalMenuCategories/AboutANA/Nursing
-Video-Gallery
https://www.youtube.com/user/RegisteredNurseRN
https://www.youtube.com/watch?v=qrBNFTv-CVE

## ■ ASSOCIATIONS

### ALZHEIMER'S ASSOCIATION
http://www.alz.org

### AMERICAN ASSOCIATION OF DIABETES EDUCATORS
www.diabeteseducator.org

### AMERICAN CANCER SOCIETY
www.cancer.org

### AMERICAN DIABETES ASSOCIATION
www.diabetes.org

### AMERICAN FOUNDATION FOR THE BLIND
http://www.afb.org/default.aspx

### AMERICAN HEART ASSOCIATION
http://www.heart.org/HEARTORG/

### AMERICAN LUNG ASSOCIATION
http://www.lung.org/

### AMERICAN NURSES ASSOCIATION
www.nursingworld.org

### ARTHRITIS FOUNDATION
www.arthritis.org

Online Resources

**BRAIN INJURY ASSOCIATION OF AMERICA**
www.biausa.org

**CYSTIC FIBROSIS FOUNDATION**
www.cff.org

**DEAFNESS RESEARCH FOUNDATION**
www.drf.org

**ENDOMETRIOSIS ASSOCIATION**
www.endometriosisassn.org

**EPILEPSY FOUNDATION**
http://www.epilepsy.com/

**HOSPICE AND PALLIATIVE NURSES ASSOCIATION**
http://advancingexpertcare.org/

**LEUKEMIA & LYMPHOMA SOCIETY**
www.lls.org/

**NATIONAL ASSOCIATION FOR CONTINENCE**
www.nafc.org

**NATIONAL ASSOCIATION FOR PRACTICAL NURSE EDUCATION AND SERVICE**
http://napnes.org/drupal-7.4/

**NATIONAL FEDERATION OF LICENSED PRACTICAL NURSES**
www.nflpn.org

**NATIONAL HEADACHE FOUNDATION**
www.headaches.org

**NATIONAL HEART, LUNG, AND BLOOD INSTITUTE**
www.nhlbi.nih.gov

**NATIONAL INSTITUTE OF ARTHRITIS AND MUSCULOSKELETAL AND SKIN DISEASES**
www.niams.nih.gov

**NATIONAL INSTITUTE ON AGING**
www.nia.nih.gov

**NATIONAL INSTITUTES OF HEALTH**
www.nih.gov

**NATIONAL KIDNEY FOUNDATION**
www.kidney.org

NATIONAL MULTIPLE SCLEROSIS SOCIETY
www.nationalmssociety.org

NATIONAL PARKINSON FOUNDATION
www.parkinson.org

NATIONAL SLEEP FOUNDATION
www.sleepfoundation.org

THE NATIONAL SPINAL CORD INJURY ASSOCIATION
www.spinalcord.org

NATIONAL STROKE ASSOCIATION
www.stroke.org

NATIONAL STUDENT NURSES ASSOCIATION
www.nsna.org

THE NORTH AMERICAN MENOPAUSE SOCIETY
www.menopause.org

PARKINSON'S DISEASE FOUNDATION
www.pdf.org

SIMON FOUNDATION FOR CONTINENCE
www.simonfoundation.org

UNITED OSTOMY ASSOCIATIONS OF AMERICA, INC
www.ostomy.org

U.S. DEPARTMENT OF HEALTH AND HUMAN SERVICES OFFICE ON
WOMEN'S HEALTH
http://www.womenshealth.gov/

## ■ DRUGS AND NUTRITION RESOURCES

DRUGS, HERBS, AND SUPPLEMENTS
http://www.accessdata.fda.gov/scripts/cder/daf/
www.cancer.gov/cancertopics/druginfo/alphalist
www.drugs.com
www.drugwatch.com
http://nccam.nih.gov/health/herbsataglance.htm
www.nlm.nih.gov/medlineplus/druginformation.html

GLUTEN-FREE DIET
http://www.mayoclinic.org/healthy-lifestyle/nutrition-and-healthy-eating
    /in-depth/gluten-free-diet/art-20048530

## LACTOSE-FREE DIET
http://www.livestrong.com/article/88755-gluten-dairy-list/

## SPECIAL DIETS AND RECIPES
www.celiac.com
www.recipesource.com/special-diets/diabetic
www.recipesource.com/special-diets/gluten-free
www.recipesource.com/special-diets/vegetarian
www.glutenfreediet.ca
www.glutenfreepassport.com
www.bestbreadrecipes.com/glutenfree.htm

## VITAMINS AND MINERALS
www.cdc.gov/nutrition/everyone/basics/vitamins
www.nlm.nih.gov/medlineplus/vitamins.html

# ■ CONTINUING EDUCATION

http://ce.nurse.com/Webinar
www.ceufast.com
www.meniscus.com/
http://www.medscape.com/nurses
http://nursingworld.org/MainMenuCategories/ThePracticeofProfessionalNursing
    /NursingEducation/ContinuingEducationforNurses
http://www.ahrq.gov/professionals/education/continuing-ed/index.html
www.rnceus.com
www.rn.org
http://www.westernschools.com/healthcare-professions/nursing

# ■ DISEASE INFORMATION

## ARTHRITIS
www.arthritis.org
www.healingwell.com/arthritis

## ASTHMA AND ALLERGIES
www.aaaai.org
www.aafa.org
http://www.mayoclinic.org/diseases-conditions/allergies/basics/definition
    /con-20034030
www.medicinenet.com/allergy/article.htm

## CANCER
www.canceradvocacy.org
www.cancer.gov
www.cancer.org
www.oncolink.org/index.cfm

## DEPRESSION
www.webmd.com/depression/default.htm
http://www.suicidepreventionlifeline.org/

## DIABETES
www.diabetes.niddk.nih.gov
www.joslin.harvard.edu

## GASTROESOPHAGEAL REFLUX DISEASE (GERD)
www.medscape.com/resource/gerd

## HEARING DIFFICULTIES
www.deaflibrary.org
http://www.hearingloss.org/content/types-causes-and-treatment

## HEPATITIS C
www.hepatitis.va.gov/
www.hepatitis-central.com/
www.hepcnet.net/
www.hcvadvocate.org/library/library.asp

## HIGH CHOLESTEROL
www.cdc.gov/cholesterol
http://www.mayoclinic.org/diseases-conditions/high-blood-cholesterol/home
    /ovc-20181871

## HIV/AIDS
www.aidsinfo.nih.gov
https://www.cdc.gov/hiv/
www.thebody.com/index/hotlines/national.html

## HOSPICE AND PALLIATIVE CARE
www.hospiceresources.net
www.growthhouse.org
www.medscape.com/resource/hospice
www.stoppain.org/palliative_care/default.asp

## HYPERTENSION
www.bplog.com/Resources.asp
http://www.nhlbi.nih.gov/health/health-topics/topics/hbp/

## INFECTION AND DISEASE CONTROL
www.cdc.gov
www.nlm.nih.gov/medlineplus/infectioncontrol.html

## LABORATORY TESTS
www.labtestsonline.org

## LOW VISION INFORMATION AND RESOURCES
www.beyondsight.com
www.lighthouse.org
www.lowvision.org

Online Resources

MIGRAINES
www.americanmigrainefoundation.org
www.headaches.org
www.healingwell.com/migraines
www.webmd.com/migraines-headaches/default.htm

PAIN
www.theacpa.org
https://www.painedu.org/resources.asp

PARKINSON DISEASE
https://www.michaeljfox.org/understanding-parkinsons/index.html?navid
    =understanding-pd
www.nlm.nih.gov/medlineplus/parkinsonsdisease.html
www.webmd.com/parkinsons-disease/default.htm

# ■ PATIENT EDUCATION

http://familydoctor.org/familydoctor/en/diseases-conditions/high-blood-pressure
    /diagnosis-tests/using-an-ambulatory-blood-pressure-monitor.html
www.ucsfhealth.org/adult/edu/index.html
https://www.nhlbi.nih.gov/health/resources/

PATIENT FINANCIAL ASSISTANCE
http://www.sutterhealth.org/about/ab_uninsured.html
http://www.patientadvocate.org/resources.php?p=482

# ■ POST-TRAUMATIC STRESS DISORDER

http://www.giftfromwithin.org/
http://www.nimh.nih.gov/health/topics/post-traumatic-stress-disorder-ptsd
    /index.shtml
http://www.ptsdalliance.org/resources.html
http://www.ptsd.va.gov/

# ■ SLEEP PROBLEMS

www.sleepassociation.org
www.sleepnet.com/insomnia2000.html
www.webmd.com/sleep-disorders/insomnia-resources

# ■ SPINE HEALTH AND BACK PROBLEMS

www.backpainreliefonline.com
www.lower-back-pain-answers.com
www.spine-health.com
www.spineuniverse.com

# ■ WOUND CARE

www.wocn.org

## ■ COMMON SEARCH ENGINES

www.ask.com
www.bing.com
www.excite.com
www.google.com
https://www.google.com/chrome/browser/
www.yahoo.com

## ■ HELP LINES AND LINKS

http://www.crisissupport.org/crisis_line
http://www.suicidepreventionlifeline.org/
http://www.dahmw.org/
http://www.helpguide.org/articles/abuse/help-for-abused-and-battered
  -women.htm
http://www.thehotline.org/blog/get-help-today/
http://www.acf.hhs.gov/programs/fysb/resource/help-fv
https://www.childhelp.org/hotline/

## ■ CUMULATIVE INDEX TO NURSING AND ALLIED HEALTH

www.ebscohost.com/academic/cinahl-plus-with-full-text/

## ■ ENGLISH-AS-SECOND LANGUAGE RESOURCES FOR NURSING STUDENTS

http://www.cabrillo.edu/academics/esl/resources.html
http://www.hospitalenglish.com/
http://nursing.gwu.edu/esl-writing-resources
http://www.usingenglish.com/links/English_for_Special_Purposes/Medical
  _English/

## ■ EVALUATION OF INTERNET RESOURCES

http://owl.english.purdue.edu/owl/resource/738/01
http://www.sc.edu/beaufort/library/pages/bones/lesson5.shtml

## ■ MEDICAL AND NURSING JOURNALS

www.nejm.org
www.jama.ama-assn.org
http://journals.lww.com/ajnonline/pages/default.aspx
www.medscape.com/welcome/journals
http://journals.lww.com/nursing/Pages/default.aspx
http://www.madeincrediblyeasy.com/products/nursing-made-incredibly-easy

## ■ NATIONAL CENTER FOR HEALTH STATISTICS

www.cdc.gov/nchs

Online Resources

## ■ TABLET AND SMARTPHONE APPLICATIONS AND SOFTWARE

http://itunes.apple.com/us/genre/mobile-software-applications/id6020?mt=8
https://apps.good.com/pce/#/apps
www.unboundmedicine.com/products

## ■ RESEARCH AND JOURNAL WEBSITES

http://www.search.com/search?q=nursing+journals
http://www.medpagetoday.com/
http://www.medscape.com/nurses

## ■ SENIOR HEALTH

http://nihseniorhealth.gov
http://www.nia.nih.gov/

## ■ UNITED STATES NATIONAL LIBRARY OF MEDICINE

www.nlm.nih.gov

# BIBLIOGRAPHY

Agency for Healthcare Research and Quality: Tool 3H: Morse Fall Scale for identifying fall risk factors. Retrieved from: http://www.ahrq.gov/professionals/systems/hospital/fallpxtoolkit/fallpxtk-tool3h.html, 2013.

Alfaro-LeFevre R: *Critical thinking, clinical reasoning, and clinical judgment: a practical approach*, ed 6, Philadelphia, 2017, Elsevier.

American Heart Association: Understanding blood pressure readings. Retrieved from: http://www.heart.org/HEARTORG/Conditions/HighBloodPressure/About HighBloodPressure/Understanding-Blood-Pressure-Readings_UCM_301764_Article.jsp#.V9Szj5grKM, August 17, 2016.

American Nurses Association: *Code of ethics for nurses with interpretive statements*, Washington, DC, 2015, American Nurses Publishing.

Bope ET, Rakel RE, Kellerman RD, editors: *Conn's current therapy 2016*, Philadelphia, 2016, Elsevier.

Brandt J, Katsma D, Crayton D, et al.: Calling in at work: acute care nursing cell phone policies, *Nurs Manage* 47(7):20–27, 2016.

Brothers K, Davis C, Kelton D, et al.: Managing your digital work life, *Nurs Made Incredibly Easy* 12(3):6–10, 2014.

Brous E: Professional licensure: investigation and disciplinary action, *AJN Am J Nurs* 112(11):53–60, 2012.

Bryant M: Cracking the code: successful strategies for studying, *Nursing2012* 42(8):16–17, 2012.

Bucks County Community College: Handouts on study skills. Retrieved from: http://www.bucks.edu/academics/tutoring/handouts/writing/readingandstudyskills/, 2016.

Chancellor J: Effective study habits for nursing students, *Nursing2013* 43(4):68–69, 2013.

Chrisman J, Jordan R, Davis C, et al.: Exploring evidence-based practice research, *Nurs Made Incredibly Easy* 12(4):8–12, 2012.

Collins SB: From "distress" to "de-stress" with stress management, *Nurse.com* 24(5):74–79, 2011.

Davis C: Keep your leadership skills sharp, *Nurs Made Incredibly Easy* 12(2):4, 2012.

Davis C: Critical thinking skills for back to school, *Nurs Made Incredibly Easy* 12(5):11–13, 2014.

Davis C, Landon D, Brothers K: Safety alert: protecting yourself and others from violence, *Nursing2015* 45(1):55–59, 2015.

deWit SC, Stromberg H, Dallred C: *Medical-surgical nursing: concepts & practice*, ed 3, St Louis, 2017, Saunders.

Dombrosky TA: Responding to verbal abuse, *Nursing2012* 42(11):58–61, 2012.

Eberhardt S: Improve handoff communication with SBAR, *Nursing2014* 44(11):17–20, 2014.

Habel M: Building nurse-physician relationships, *Nurse.com* 25(6):28–33, 2012.

Hanna AF, Suplee PD: Don't cross the line: respecting professional boundaries, *Nursing2012* 42(9):41–47, 2012.

Hart TL: *Speedy Spanish for medical personnel*, Santa Barbara, CA, 1980, Baja Books.

Hart TL: *Speedy Spanish for nursing personnel*, Santa Barbara, CA, 1988, Baja Books.

Haugh KH: Head-to-toe: organizing your baseline patient physical assessment, *Nursing2015* 45(12):58–61, 2015.

High-alert medications: no margin for error, *Nursing2012* 42(8):10, 2012.

Hill SS, Howlett HS: *Success in practical/vocational nursing: from student to leader*, ed 7, St Louis, 2012, Saunders.

Ignatavicius DD, Workman ML: *Medical-surgical nursing: critical thinking for collaborative care*, ed 8, St Louis, 2016, Elsevier.

*Institute for Safe Medication Practices: ISMP's list of error-prone abbreviations, symbols, and dose designations.* Retrieved from: http://www.ismp.org/tools/errorproneabbreviations.pdf, 2015.

Joyce EV, Villanueva ME: *Say it in Spanish: a guide for health care professionals*, ed 3, Philadelphia, 2004, Saunders.

Kee J, Hayes E, McCuistion L: *Pharmacology: a patient-centered nursing process approach*, ed 8, St Louis, 2015, Elsevier.

Kirchner RB: Introducing nursing informatics, *Nursing2014* 44(9):22–23, 2014.

Lamos EM, Younk LM, Davis SN: Concentrated insulins: the new basal insulins, *Ther Clin Risk Manag* 12: 389–400, 2016.

Lange C: Nursing and the importance of body language, *Nursing2016* 46(4):48–49, 2016.

Langford RW: *Mosby's PDQ for LPN*, ed 3, St Louis, 2013, Elsevier.

Laskowski-Jones L: The art of harmonious delegation, *Nursing2014* 44(5):6, 2014.

Lee A: The role of informatics in nursing, *Nurs Made Incredibly Easy* 12(4):55, 2014.

Lewis SL, Bucher L, Heitkemper MM, et al.: *Medical-surgical nursing: assessment & management of clinical problems*, ed 9, St Louis, 2014, Mosby.

Mahan LK, Raymond JL: *Krause's food, nutrition, & diet therapy*, ed 14, St Louis, 2017, Mosby.

Mattison M: Hospital management of older adults. Retrieved from: https://www.uptodate.com/contents/hospital-management-of-older-adults?source=search_result&search=hospital+management+of+older+adults&selected Title=1%7E150, 2016.

Mayo Clinic Staff: Post-traumatic stress disorder (PTSD). Retrieved from: http://www.mayoclinic.org/diseases-conditions/post-traumatic-stress-disorder/basics/definition/con-20022540, 2014.

McBride S, Delaney JM, Tietze M: Health information technology and nursing, *AJN Am J Nurs* 112(8):36–42, 2012.

McCarron K: Routine labs for common meds, *Nurs Made Incredibly Easy* 11(2):50–53, 2013.

Merritt S: Tips for computer-based multiple choice tests (CBT, CBE, and CAT). Retrieved from: http://masteringmultiple choice.com/2009/09/tips-for-computer-based-multiple-choice-tests-cbt-cbe-and-cat/, 2009.

Miadowicz H: Biofeedback 101, *Nurse.com* 27(11):44–49, 2014.

National Institute of Mental Health: Post-traumatic stress disorder. Retrieved from: http://www.nimh.nih.gov/health/topics/post-traumatic-stress-disorder-ptsd/index.shtml, 2016.

Nugent PM, Vitale BA: *Test success: test-taking techniques for beginning nursing students*, ed 6, Philadelphia, 2012, FA Davis.

Nursing2013 Editors: Getting a grip on stress, *Nurse.com* 43(6):40, 2013.

Ortega L, Parsh B: Improving change-of-shift report, *Nursing2013* 43(2):68, 2013.

O'Toole MT, editor: *Mosby's dictionary of medicine, nursing & health professions*, ed 10, St Louis, 2017, Mosby.

Pagana KD: New Nurse Notes: 7 tips to improve your professional etiquette, *OR Nurse* 4(2):14–17, 2010.

Pagana KD: Facebook: know the policy before posting, *Nurse.com* 24(6):55–59, 2012.

Pagana KD: Mind your manners … multi-culturally, *Nurse.com* 24(6):49–51, 2012.

Pasero C, McCaffery M: *Pain assessment and pharmacologic management*, St Louis, 2011, Mosby.

Pauk W, Owens RJQ: *How to study in college*, ed 11, New York, 2014, Cengage Learning.

Peckenpaugh NJ, Poleman CM: *Nutrition essentials and diet therapy*, ed 11, Philadelphia, 2010, Saunders.

Penn State Division of Undergraduate Studies: Study skills. Retrieved from: http://dus.psu.edu/academicsuccess/studyskills.html, 2014.

Phillips S: Foods to avoid with lactose intolerance. Retrieved from: http://www.livestrong.com/article/70598-lactose-intolerance-foods-avoid/, 2015. Accessed September 24, 2016.

Piscotty R, Voepel-Lewis T, Lee S, et al.: Hold the phone? Nurses, social media and patient care, *Nursing2015* 45(5): 64–67, 2015.

Potter PA, Perry AG, Ostendorf W: *Clinical nursing skills & techniques*, ed 8, St Louis, 2014, Mosby.

Potter PA, Perry AG, Stockert PA, et al.: *Fundamentals of nursing*, ed 9, St Louis, 2017, Mosby.

Rosati LJ: Strike gold when interviewing for your first nursing job, *Nursing2014* 44(5):49–52, 2014.

Sherman RO: Evidence-based effective nursing leadership, *Nurse.com* 25(5): 68–73, 2012.

Nursing Matters: SMART goals. Retrieved from: http://nursing-matters.com/smart-goals/, 2016.

Smith LS: How to finance your dreams of further education. In *Lippincott's 2012 Nursing Career Directory*, Philadelphia, 2012, Wolters Kluwer/Lippincott Williams & Wilkins, pp 28–33.

Strickler J: When it hurts to care: work-place violence in healthcare, *Nursing2013* 43(4):58–62, 2013.

Taylor S: Research reveals the benefits of meditation, *Nurse.com* 27(10):36–41, 2014.

Texas Crime Watch: Rape: ideas for self-protection (pamphlet), n.d., Austin, Texas.

Truven Health Analytics Inc: Gluten-free diet: aftercare instructions. Retrieved from http://www.drugs.com/cg/gluten-free-diet-aftercare-instructions.html, 2015.

Tubesing DA: *Kicking your stress habits*, New York, 1992, Penguin Group.

Ulrich D, Stalter A: Securing your first clinical nursing position, *Nursing* 45(8):60–63, 2015.

University of North Carolina Greensboro. http://learn-more.uncg.edu/blog/bid/157637/Success-Tips-for-Taking-Online-Exams, 2014.

U.S. Department of Health and Human Services and U.S. Department of Agriculture: Dietary Guidelines for Americans 2015–2020, ed 8. Available at: http://health.gov/dietaryguidelines/2015/guidelines/.

Williams P: *Fundamental concepts and skills for nursing*, ed 5, St Louis, 2018, Saunders.

Williams SG: Back to school, *Advance for Nurses* 8(3):22–23, 2011.

Woods AD: Implementing evidence into practice. Lippincott's 2013 Nursing Career & Education Directory, *Nursing2013* 43(1 suppl):4–6, 2013.

Zerwekh J, Garneau AZ: *Nursing today: transition and trends*, ed 8, Philadelphia, 2015, Saunders.

# MAY 2017

| SUNDAY | MONDAY | TUESDAY | WEDNESDAY | THURSDAY | FRIDAY | SATURDAY |
|--------|--------|---------|-----------|----------|--------|----------|
|        | 1      | 2       | 3         | 4        | 5      | 6        |
| 7      | 8      | 9       | 10        | 11       | 12     | 13       |
| 14     | 15     | 16      | 17        | 18       | 19     | 20       |
| 21     | 22     | 23      | 24        | 25       | 26     | 27       |
| 28     | 29     | 30      | 31        |          |        |          |

# JUNE 2017

| SUNDAY | MONDAY | TUESDAY | WEDNESDAY | THURSDAY | FRIDAY | SATURDAY |
|--------|--------|---------|-----------|----------|--------|----------|
|        |        |         |           | 1        | 2      | 3        |
| 4      | 5      | 6       | 7         | 8        | 9      | 10       |
| 11     | 12     | 13      | 14        | 15       | 16     | 17       |
| 18     | 19     | 20      | 21        | 22       | 23     | 24       |
| 25     | 26     | 27      | 28        | 29       | 30     |          |

# JULY 2017

| SUNDAY | MONDAY | TUESDAY | WEDNESDAY | THURSDAY | FRIDAY | SATURDAY |
|--------|--------|---------|-----------|----------|--------|----------|
|        |        |         |           |          |        | 1        |
| 2      | 3      | 4       | 5         | 6        | 7      | 8        |
| 9      | 10     | 11      | 12        | 13       | 14     | 15       |
| 16     | 17     | 18      | 19        | 20       | 21     | 22       |
| 23     | 24     | 25      | 26        | 27       | 28     | 29       |
| 30     | 31     |         |           |          |        |          |

# AUGUST 2017

| SUNDAY | MONDAY | TUESDAY | WEDNESDAY | THURSDAY | FRIDAY | SATURDAY |
|--------|--------|---------|-----------|----------|--------|----------|
|        |        | 1       | 2         | 3        | 4      | 5        |
| 6      | 7      | 8       | 9         | 10       | 11     | 12       |
| 13     | 14     | 15      | 16        | 17       | 18     | 19       |
| 20     | 21     | 22      | 23        | 24       | 25     | 26       |
| 27     | 28     | 29      | 30        | 31       |        |          |

# SEPTEMBER 2017

| SUNDAY | MONDAY | TUESDAY | WEDNESDAY | THURSDAY | FRIDAY | SATURDAY |
|--------|--------|---------|-----------|----------|--------|----------|
|        |        |         |           |          | 1      | 2        |
| 3      | 4      | 5       | 6         | 7        | 8      | 9        |
| 10     | 11     | 12      | 13        | 14       | 15     | 16       |
| 17     | 18     | 19      | 20        | 21       | 22     | 23       |
| 24     | 25     | 26      | 27        | 28       | 29     | 30       |

# OCTOBER 2017

| SUNDAY | MONDAY | TUESDAY | WEDNESDAY | THURSDAY | FRIDAY | SATURDAY |
|--------|--------|---------|-----------|----------|--------|----------|
| 1 | 2 | 3 | 4 | 5 | 6 | 7 |
| 8 | 9 | 10 | 11 | 12 | 13 | 14 |
| 15 | 16 | 17 | 18 | 19 | 20 | 21 |
| 22 | 23 | 24 | 25 | 26 | 27 | 28 |
| 29 | 30 | 31 | | | | |

# NOVEMBER 2017

| SUNDAY | MONDAY | TUESDAY | WEDNESDAY | THURSDAY | FRIDAY | SATURDAY |
|--------|--------|---------|-----------|----------|--------|----------|
|        |        |         | 1         | 2        | 3      | 4        |
| 5      | 6      | 7       | 8         | 9        | 10     | 11       |
| 12     | 13     | 14      | 15        | 16       | 17     | 18       |
| 19     | 20     | 21      | 22        | 23       | 24     | 25       |
| 26     | 27     | 28      | 29        | 30       |        |          |

# DECEMBER 2017

| SUNDAY | MONDAY | TUESDAY | WEDNESDAY | THURSDAY | FRIDAY | SATURDAY |
|--------|--------|---------|-----------|----------|--------|----------|
|  |  |  |  |  | 1 | 2 |
| 3 | 4 | 5 | 6 | 7 | 8 | 9 |
| 10 | 11 | 12 | 13 | 14 | 15 | 16 |
| 17 | 18 | 19 | 20 | 21 | 22 | 23 |
| 24 | 25 | 26 | 27 | 28 | 29 | 30 |
| 31 |  |  |  |  |  |  |

Monthly Calendar

# JANUARY 2018

| SUNDAY | MONDAY | TUESDAY | WEDNESDAY | THURSDAY | FRIDAY | SATURDAY |
|--------|--------|---------|-----------|----------|--------|----------|
|        | 1      | 2       | 3         | 4        | 5      | 6        |
| 7      | 8      | 9       | 10        | 11       | 12     | 13       |
| 14     | 15     | 16      | 17        | 18       | 19     | 20       |
| 21     | 22     | 23      | 24        | 25       | 26     | 27       |
| 28     | 29     | 30      | 31        |          |        |          |

# FEBRUARY 2018

| SUNDAY | MONDAY | TUESDAY | WEDNESDAY | THURSDAY | FRIDAY | SATURDAY |
|--------|--------|---------|-----------|----------|--------|----------|
|        |        |         |           | 1        | 2      | 3        |
| 4      | 5      | 6       | 7         | 8        | 9      | 10       |
| 11     | 12     | 13      | 14        | 15       | 16     | 17       |
| 18     | 19     | 20      | 21        | 22       | 23     | 24       |
| 25     | 26     | 27      | 28        |          |        |          |

Monthly Calendar

# MARCH 2018

| SUNDAY | MONDAY | TUESDAY | WEDNESDAY | THURSDAY | FRIDAY | SATURDAY |
|--------|--------|---------|-----------|----------|--------|----------|
|        |        |         |           | 1        | 2      | 3        |
| 4      | 5      | 6       | 7         | 8        | 9      | 10       |
| 11     | 12     | 13      | 14        | 15       | 16     | 17       |
| 18     | 19     | 20      | 21        | 22       | 23     | 24       |
| 25     | 26     | 27      | 28        | 29       | 30     | 31       |

# APRIL 2018

| SUNDAY | MONDAY | TUESDAY | WEDNESDAY | THURSDAY | FRIDAY | SATURDAY |
|--------|--------|---------|-----------|----------|--------|----------|
| 1 | 2 | 3 | 4 | 5 | 6 | 7 |
| 8 | 9 | 10 | 11 | 12 | 13 | 14 |
| 15 | 16 | 17 | 18 | 19 | 20 | 21 |
| 22 | 23 | 24 | 25 | 26 | 27 | 28 |
| 29 | 30 | | | | | |

# MAY 2018

| SUNDAY | MONDAY | TUESDAY | WEDNESDAY | THURSDAY | FRIDAY | SATURDAY |
|--------|--------|---------|-----------|----------|--------|----------|
|        |        | 1       | 2         | 3        | 4      | 5        |
| 6      | 7      | 8       | 9         | 10       | 11     | 12       |
| 13     | 14     | 15      | 16        | 17       | 18     | 19       |
| 20     | 21     | 22      | 23        | 24       | 25     | 26       |
| 27     | 28     | 29      | 30        | 31       |        |          |

# JUNE 2018

| SUNDAY | MONDAY | TUESDAY | WEDNESDAY | THURSDAY | FRIDAY | SATURDAY |
|--------|--------|---------|-----------|----------|--------|----------|
|        |        |         |           |          | 1      | 2        |
| 3      | 4      | 5       | 6         | 7        | 8      | 9        |
| 10     | 11     | 12      | 13        | 14       | 15     | 16       |
| 17     | 18     | 19      | 20        | 21       | 22     | 23       |
| 24     | 25     | 26      | 27        | 28       | 29     | 30       |

# JULY 2018

| SUNDAY | MONDAY | TUESDAY | WEDNESDAY | THURSDAY | FRIDAY | SATURDAY |
|--------|--------|---------|-----------|----------|--------|----------|
| 1 | 2 | 3 | 4 | 5 | 6 | 7 |
| 8 | 9 | 10 | 11 | 12 | 13 | 14 |
| 15 | 16 | 17 | 18 | 19 | 20 | 21 |
| 22 | 23 | 24 | 25 | 26 | 27 | 28 |
| 29 | 30 | 31 | | | | |

# AUGUST 2018

| SUNDAY | MONDAY | TUESDAY | WEDNESDAY | THURSDAY | FRIDAY | SATURDAY |
|--------|--------|---------|-----------|----------|--------|----------|
|        |        |         | 1         | 2        | 3      | 4        |
| 5      | 6      | 7       | 8         | 9        | 10     | 11       |
| 12     | 13     | 14      | 15        | 16       | 17     | 18       |
| 19     | 20     | 21      | 22        | 23       | 24     | 25       |
| 26     | 27     | 28      | 29        | 30       | 31     |          |

# SEPTEMBER 2018

| SUNDAY | MONDAY | TUESDAY | WEDNESDAY | THURSDAY | FRIDAY | SATURDAY |
|--------|--------|---------|-----------|----------|--------|----------|
|        |        |         |           |          |        | 1        |
| 2      | 3      | 4       | 5         | 6        | 7      | 8        |
| 9      | 10     | 11      | 12        | 13       | 14     | 15       |
| 16     | 17     | 18      | 19        | 20       | 21     | 22       |
| 23     | 24     | 25      | 26        | 27       | 28     | 29       |
| 30     |        |         |           |          |        |          |

# OCTOBER 2018

| SUNDAY | MONDAY | TUESDAY | WEDNESDAY | THURSDAY | FRIDAY | SATURDAY |
|--------|--------|---------|-----------|----------|--------|----------|
|        | 1      | 2       | 3         | 4        | 5      | 6        |
| 7      | 8      | 9       | 10        | 11       | 12     | 13       |
| 14     | 15     | 16      | 17        | 18       | 19     | 20       |
| 21     | 22     | 23      | 24        | 25       | 26     | 27       |
| 28     | 29     | 30      | 31        |          |        |          |

# NOVEMBER 2018

| SUNDAY | MONDAY | TUESDAY | WEDNESDAY | THURSDAY | FRIDAY | SATURDAY |
|--------|--------|---------|-----------|----------|--------|----------|
|        |        |         |           | 1        | 2      | 3        |
| 4      | 5      | 6       | 7         | 8        | 9      | 10       |
| 11     | 12     | 13      | 14        | 15       | 16     | 17       |
| 18     | 19     | 20      | 21        | 22       | 23     | 24       |
| 25     | 26     | 27      | 28        | 29       | 30     |          |

# DECEMBER 2018

| SUNDAY | MONDAY | TUESDAY | WEDNESDAY | THURSDAY | FRIDAY | SATURDAY |
|--------|--------|---------|-----------|----------|--------|----------|
| | | | | | | 1 |
| 2 | 3 | 4 | 5 | 6 | 7 | 8 |
| 9 | 10 | 11 | 12 | 13 | 14 | 15 |
| 16 | 17 | 18 | 19 | 20 | 21 | 22 |
| 23 | 24 | 25 | 26 | 27 | 28 | 29 |
| 30 | 31 | | | | | |

MONDAY **MAY 1**

TUESDAY **MAY 2**

WEDNESDAY **MAY 3**

THURSDAY **MAY 4**

FRIDAY **MAY 5**

SATURDAY **MAY 6**

SUNDAY **MAY 7**

MONDAY **MAY 8**

TUESDAY **MAY 9**

WEDNESDAY **MAY 10**

THURSDAY **MAY 11**

FRIDAY **MAY 12**

SATURDAY **MAY 13**

SUNDAY **MAY 14**

Weekly Planner

MONDAY **MAY 15**

TUESDAY **MAY 16**

WEDNESDAY **MAY 17**

THURSDAY **MAY 18**

FRIDAY **MAY 19**

SATURDAY **MAY 20**

SUNDAY **MAY 21**

MONDAY **MAY 22**

TUESDAY **MAY 23**

WEDNESDAY **MAY 24**

THURSDAY **MAY 25**

FRIDAY **MAY 26**

SATURDAY **MAY 27**

SUNDAY **MAY 28**

Weekly Planner

MONDAY **MAY 29**

TUESDAY **MAY 30**

WEDNESDAY **MAY 31**

THURSDAY **JUNE 1**

FRIDAY **JUNE 2**

SATURDAY **JUNE 3**

SUNDAY **JUNE 4**

## MONDAY JUNE 5

## TUESDAY JUNE 6

## WEDNESDAY JUNE 7

## THURSDAY JUNE 8

## FRIDAY JUNE 9

## SATURDAY JUNE 10

## SUNDAY JUNE 11

Weekly Planner

MONDAY **JUNE 12**

TUESDAY **JUNE 13**

WEDNESDAY **JUNE 14**

THURSDAY **JUNE 15**

FRIDAY **JUNE 16**

SATURDAY **JUNE 17**

SUNDAY **JUNE 18**

MONDAY **JUNE 19**

TUESDAY **JUNE 20**

WEDNESDAY **JUNE 21**

THURSDAY **JUNE 22**

FRIDAY **JUNE 23**

SATURDAY **JUNE 24**

SUNDAY **JUNE 25**

Weekly Planner

MONDAY **JUNE 26**

TUESDAY **JUNE 27**

WEDNESDAY **JUNE 28**

THURSDAY **JUNE 29**

FRIDAY **JUNE 30**

SATURDAY **JULY 1**

SUNDAY **JULY 2**

# JULY 3-9

MONDAY **JULY 3**

TUESDAY **JULY 4**

WEDNESDAY **JULY 5**

THURSDAY **JULY 6**

FRIDAY **JULY 7**

SATURDAY **JULY 8**

SUNDAY **JULY 9**

## MONDAY **JULY 10**

## TUESDAY **JULY 11**

## WEDNESDAY **JULY 12**

## THURSDAY **JULY 13**

## FRIDAY **JULY 14**

## SATURDAY **JULY 15**

## SUNDAY **JULY 16**

## MONDAY JULY 17

## TUESDAY JULY 18

## WEDNESDAY JULY 19

## THURSDAY JULY 20

## FRIDAY JULY 21

## SATURDAY JULY 22

## SUNDAY JULY 23

MONDAY **JULY 24**

TUESDAY **JULY 25**

WEDNESDAY **JULY 26**

THURSDAY **JULY 27**

FRIDAY **JULY 28**

SATURDAY **JULY 29**

SUNDAY **JULY 30**

MONDAY **JULY 31**

TUESDAY **AUGUST 1**

WEDNESDAY **AUGUST 2**

THURSDAY **AUGUST 3**

FRIDAY **AUGUST 4**

SATURDAY **AUGUST 5**

SUNDAY **AUGUST 6**

Weekly Planner

# AUGUST 7-13          2017

**MONDAY AUGUST 7**

**TUESDAY AUGUST 8**

**WEDNESDAY AUGUST 9**

**THURSDAY AUGUST 10**

**FRIDAY AUGUST 11**

**SATURDAY AUGUST 12**

**SUNDAY AUGUST 13**

MONDAY **AUGUST 14**

TUESDAY **AUGUST 15**

WEDNESDAY **AUGUST 16**

THURSDAY **AUGUST 17**

FRIDAY **AUGUST 18**

SATURDAY **AUGUST 19**

SUNDAY **AUGUST 20**

Weekly Planner

# AUGUST 21-27 2017

MONDAY **AUGUST 21**

TUESDAY **AUGUST 22**

WEDNESDAY **AUGUST 23**

THURSDAY **AUGUST 24**

FRIDAY **AUGUST 25**

SATURDAY **AUGUST 26**

SUNDAY **AUGUST 27**

MONDAY **AUGUST 28**

TUESDAY **AUGUST 29**

WEDNESDAY **AUGUST 30**

THURSDAY **AUGUST 31**

FRIDAY **SEPTEMBER 1**

SATURDAY **SEPTEMBER 2**

SUNDAY **SEPTEMBER 3**

Weekly Planner

# SEPTEMBER 4-10 2017

MONDAY **SEPTEMBER 4**

TUESDAY **SEPTEMBER 5**

WEDNESDAY **SEPTEMBER 6**

THURSDAY **SEPTEMBER 7**

FRIDAY **SEPTEMBER 8**

SATURDAY **SEPTEMBER 9**

SUNDAY **SEPTEMBER 10**

# SEPTEMBER 11-17 2017

MONDAY **SEPTEMBER 11**

TUESDAY **SEPTEMBER 12**

WEDNESDAY **SEPTEMBER 13**

THURSDAY **SEPTEMBER 14**

FRIDAY **SEPTEMBER 15**

SATURDAY **SEPTEMBER 16**

SUNDAY **SEPTEMBER 17**

# SEPTEMBER 18-24 2017

MONDAY **SEPTEMBER 18**

TUESDAY **SEPTEMBER 19**

WEDNESDAY **SEPTEMBER 20**

THURSDAY **SEPTEMBER 21**

FRIDAY **SEPTEMBER 22**

SATURDAY **SEPTEMBER 23**

SUNDAY **SEPTEMBER 24**

MONDAY **SEPTEMBER 25**

TUESDAY **SEPTEMBER 26**

WEDNESDAY **SEPTEMBER 27**

THURSDAY **SEPTEMBER 28**

FRIDAY **SEPTEMBER 29**

SATURDAY **SEPTEMBER 30**

SUNDAY **OCTOBER 1**

Weekly Planner

MONDAY **OCTOBER 2**

TUESDAY **OCTOBER 3**

WEDNESDAY **OCTOBER 4**

THURSDAY **OCTOBER 5**

FRIDAY **OCTOBER 6**

SATURDAY **OCTOBER 7**

SUNDAY **OCTOBER 8**

MONDAY **OCTOBER 9**

TUESDAY **OCTOBER 10**

WEDNESDAY **OCTOBER 11**

THURSDAY **OCTOBER 12**

FRIDAY **OCTOBER 13**

SATURDAY **OCTOBER 14**

SUNDAY **OCTOBER 15**

Weekly Planner

# OCTOBER 16-22 2017

MONDAY **OCTOBER 16**

TUESDAY **OCTOBER 17**

WEDNESDAY **OCTOBER 18**

THURSDAY **OCTOBER 19**

FRIDAY **OCTOBER 20**

SATURDAY **OCTOBER 21**

SUNDAY **OCTOBER 22**

# OCTOBER 23-29 2017

## MONDAY OCTOBER 23

## TUESDAY OCTOBER 24

## WEDNESDAY OCTOBER 25

## THURSDAY OCTOBER 26

## FRIDAY OCTOBER 27

## SATURDAY OCTOBER 28

## SUNDAY OCTOBER 29

# OCT 30-NOV 5 2017

MONDAY **OCTOBER 30**

TUESDAY **OCTOBER 31**

WEDNESDAY **NOVEMBER 1**

THURSDAY **NOVEMBER 2**

FRIDAY **NOVEMBER 3**

SATURDAY **NOVEMBER 4**

SUNDAY **NOVEMBER 5**

MONDAY **NOVEMBER 6**

TUESDAY **NOVEMBER 7**

WEDNESDAY **NOVEMBER 8**

THURSDAY **NOVEMBER 9**

FRIDAY **NOVEMBER 10**

SATURDAY **NOVEMBER 11**

SUNDAY **NOVEMBER 12**

Weekly Planner

# NOVEMBER 13-19

**MONDAY NOVEMBER 13**

**TUESDAY NOVEMBER 14**

**WEDNESDAY NOVEMBER 15**

**THURSDAY NOVEMBER 16**

**FRIDAY NOVEMBER 17**

**SATURDAY NOVEMBER 18**

**SUNDAY NOVEMBER 19**

MONDAY **NOVEMBER 20**

TUESDAY **NOVEMBER 21**

WEDNESDAY **NOVEMBER 22**

THURSDAY **NOVEMBER 23**

FRIDAY **NOVEMBER 24**

SATURDAY **NOVEMBER 25**

SUNDAY **NOVEMBER 26**

Weekly Planner

MONDAY **NOVEMBER 27**

TUESDAY **NOVEMBER 28**

WEDNESDAY **NOVEMBER 29**

THURSDAY **NOVEMBER 30**

FRIDAY **DECEMBER 1**

SATURDAY **DECEMBER 2**

SUNDAY **DECEMBER 3**

# DECEMBER 4-10                    2017

## MONDAY DECEMBER 4

## TUESDAY DECEMBER 5

## WEDNESDAY DECEMBER 6

## THURSDAY DECEMBER 7

## FRIDAY DECEMBER 8

## SATURDAY DECEMBER 9

## SUNDAY DECEMBER 10

MONDAY **DECEMBER 11**

TUESDAY **DECEMBER 12**

WEDNESDAY **DECEMBER 13**

THURSDAY **DECEMBER 14**

FRIDAY **DECEMBER 15**

SATURDAY **DECEMBER 16**

SUNDAY **DECEMBER 17**

# DECEMBER 18-24     2017

MONDAY **DECEMBER 18**

TUESDAY **DECEMBER 19**

WEDNESDAY **DECEMBER 20**

THURSDAY **DECEMBER 21**

FRIDAY **DECEMBER 22**

SATURDAY **DECEMBER 23**

SUNDAY **DECEMBER 24**

MONDAY **DECEMBER 25**

TUESDAY **DECEMBER 26**

WEDNESDAY **DECEMBER 27**

THURSDAY **DECEMBER 28**

FRIDAY **DECEMBER 29**

SATURDAY **DECEMBER 30**

SUNDAY **DECEMBER 31**

MONDAY **JANUARY 1**

TUESDAY **JANUARY 2**

WEDNESDAY **JANUARY 3**

THURSDAY **JANUARY 4**

FRIDAY **JANUARY 5**

SATURDAY **JANUARY 6**

SUNDAY **JANUARY 7**

MONDAY **JANUARY 8**

TUESDAY **JANUARY 9**

WEDNESDAY **JANUARY 10**

THURSDAY **JANUARY 11**

FRIDAY **JANUARY 12**

SATURDAY **JANUARY 13**

SUNDAY **JANUARY 14**

MONDAY **JANUARY 15**

TUESDAY **JANUARY 16**

WEDNESDAY **JANUARY 17**

THURSDAY **JANUARY 18**

FRIDAY **JANUARY 19**

SATURDAY **JANUARY 20**

SUNDAY **JANUARY 21**

Weekly Planner

# JANUARY 22-28　　2018

MONDAY **JANUARY 22**

TUESDAY **JANUARY 23**

WEDNESDAY **JANUARY 24**

THURSDAY **JANUARY 25**

FRIDAY **JANUARY 26**

SATURDAY **JANUARY 27**

SUNDAY **JANUARY 28**

## MONDAY JANUARY 29

## TUESDAY JANUARY 30

## WEDNESDAY JANUARY 31

## THURSDAY FEBRUARY 1

## FRIDAY FEBRUARY 2

## SATURDAY FEBRUARY 3

## SUNDAY FEBRUARY 4

# FEBRUARY 5-11                    2018

MONDAY **FEBRUARY 5**

TUESDAY **FEBRUARY 6**

WEDNESDAY **FEBRUARY 7**

THURSDAY **FEBRUARY 8**

FRIDAY **FEBRUARY 9**

SATURDAY **FEBRUARY 10**

SUNDAY **FEBRUARY 11**

MONDAY **FEBRUARY 12**

TUESDAY **FEBRUARY 13**

WEDNESDAY **FEBRUARY 14**

THURSDAY **FEBRUARY 15**

FRIDAY **FEBRUARY 16**

SATURDAY **FEBRUARY 17**

SUNDAY **FEBRUARY 18**

Weekly Planner

# FEBRUARY 19-25 2018

MONDAY **FEBRUARY 19**

TUESDAY **FEBRUARY 20**

WEDNESDAY **FEBRUARY 21**

THURSDAY **FEBRUARY 22**

FRIDAY **FEBRUARY 23**

SATURDAY **FEBRUARY 24**

SUNDAY **FEBRUARY 25**

MONDAY **FEBRUARY 26**

TUESDAY **FEBRUARY 27**

WEDNESDAY **FEBRUARY 28**

THURSDAY **MARCH 1**

FRIDAY **MARCH 2**

SATURDAY **MARCH 3**

SUNDAY **MARCH 4**

Weekly Planner

# MARCH 5-11 2018

MONDAY **MARCH 5**

TUESDAY **MARCH 6**

WEDNESDAY **MARCH 7**

THURSDAY **MARCH 8**

FRIDAY **MARCH 9**

SATURDAY **MARCH 10**

SUNDAY **MARCH 11**

MONDAY **MARCH 12**

TUESDAY **MARCH 13**

WEDNESDAY **MARCH 14**

THURSDAY **MARCH 15**

FRIDAY **MARCH 16**

SATURDAY **MARCH 17**

SUNDAY **MARCH 18**

Weekly Planner

# MARCH 19-25 2018

MONDAY **MARCH 19**

TUESDAY **MARCH 20**

WEDNESDAY **MARCH 21**

THURSDAY **MARCH 22**

FRIDAY **MARCH 23**

SATURDAY **MARCH 24**

SUNDAY **MARCH 25**

MONDAY **MARCH 26**

TUESDAY **MARCH 27**

WEDNESDAY **MARCH 28**

THURSDAY **MARCH 29**

FRIDAY **MARCH 30**

SATURDAY **MARCH 31**

SUNDAY **APRIL 1**

Weekly Planner

MONDAY **APRIL 2**

TUESDAY **APRIL 3**

WEDNESDAY **APRIL 4**

THURSDAY **APRIL 5**

FRIDAY **APRIL 6**

SATURDAY **APRIL 7**

SUNDAY **APRIL 8**

MONDAY **APRIL 9**

TUESDAY **APRIL 10**

WEDNESDAY **APRIL 11**

THURSDAY **APRIL 12**

FRIDAY **APRIL 13**

SATURDAY **APRIL 14**

SUNDAY **APRIL 15**

Weekly Planner

# APRIL 16-22　　　　　　2018

MONDAY **APRIL 16**

TUESDAY **APRIL 17**

WEDNESDAY **APRIL 18**

THURSDAY **APRIL 19**

FRIDAY **APRIL 20**

SATURDAY **APRIL 21**　　　　　SUNDAY **APRIL 22**

MONDAY **APRIL 23**

TUESDAY **APRIL 24**

WEDNESDAY **APRIL 25**

THURSDAY **APRIL 26**

FRIDAY **APRIL 27**

SATURDAY **APRIL 28**

SUNDAY **APRIL 29**

MONDAY **APRIL 30**

TUESDAY **MAY 1**

WEDNESDAY **MAY 2**

THURSDAY **MAY 3**

FRIDAY **MAY 4**

SATURDAY **MAY 5**

SUNDAY **MAY 6**

## MONDAY **MAY 7**

## TUESDAY **MAY 8**

## WEDNESDAY **MAY 9**

## THURSDAY **MAY 10**

## FRIDAY **MAY 11**

## SATURDAY **MAY 12**

## SUNDAY **MAY 13**

## MONDAY **MAY 14**

## TUESDAY **MAY 15**

## WEDNESDAY **MAY 16**

## THURSDAY **MAY 17**

## FRIDAY **MAY 18**

## SATURDAY **MAY 19**

## SUNDAY **MAY 20**

# MAY 21-27

MONDAY **MAY 21**

TUESDAY **MAY 22**

WEDNESDAY **MAY 23**

THURSDAY **MAY 24**

FRIDAY **MAY 25**

SATURDAY **MAY 26**

SUNDAY **MAY 27**

Weekly Planner

MONDAY **MAY 28**

TUESDAY **MAY 29**

WEDNESDAY **MAY 30**

THURSDAY **MAY 31**

FRIDAY **JUNE 1**

SATURDAY **JUNE 2**

SUNDAY **JUNE 3**

MONDAY **JUNE 4**

TUESDAY **JUNE 5**

WEDNESDAY **JUNE 6**

THURSDAY **JUNE 7**

FRIDAY **JUNE 8**

SATURDAY **JUNE 9**

SUNDAY **JUNE 10**

Weekly Planner

## JUNE 11-17 2018

MONDAY **JUNE 11**

TUESDAY **JUNE 12**

WEDNESDAY **JUNE 13**

THURSDAY **JUNE 14**

FRIDAY **JUNE 15**

SATURDAY **JUNE 16**

SUNDAY **JUNE 17**

# JUNE 18-24                                    2018

## MONDAY JUNE 18

## TUESDAY JUNE 19

## WEDNESDAY JUNE 20

## THURSDAY JUNE 21

## FRIDAY JUNE 22

## SATURDAY JUNE 23

## SUNDAY JUNE 24

MONDAY **JUNE 25**

TUESDAY **JUNE 26**

WEDNESDAY **JUNE 27**

THURSDAY **JUNE 28**

FRIDAY **JUNE 29**

SATURDAY **JUNE 30**

SUNDAY **JULY I**

# JULY 2-8 2018

## MONDAY JULY 2

## TUESDAY JULY 3

## WEDNESDAY JULY 4

## THURSDAY JULY 5

## FRIDAY JULY 6

## SATURDAY JULY 7

## SUNDAY JULY 8

Weekly Planner

MONDAY **JULY 9**

TUESDAY **JULY 10**

WEDNESDAY **JULY 11**

THURSDAY **JULY 12**

FRIDAY **JULY 13**

SATURDAY **JULY 14**

SUNDAY **JULY 15**

# JULY 16-22 2018

## MONDAY JULY 16

## TUESDAY JULY 17

## WEDNESDAY JULY 18

## THURSDAY JULY 19

## FRIDAY JULY 20

## SATURDAY JULY 21

## SUNDAY JULY 22

Weekly Planner

# JULY 23-29

**MONDAY JULY 23**

**TUESDAY JULY 24**

**WEDNESDAY JULY 25**

**THURSDAY JULY 26**

**FRIDAY JULY 27**

**SATURDAY JULY 28**

**SUNDAY JULY 29**

MONDAY **JULY 30**

TUESDAY **JULY 31**

WEDNESDAY **AUGUST 1**

THURSDAY **AUGUST 2**

FRIDAY **AUGUST 3**

SATURDAY **AUGUST 4**

SUNDAY **AUGUST 5**

Weekly Planner

MONDAY **AUGUST 6**

TUESDAY **AUGUST 7**

WEDNESDAY **AUGUST 8**

THURSDAY **AUGUST 9**

FRIDAY **AUGUST 10**

SATURDAY **AUGUST 11**

SUNDAY **AUGUST 12**

### MONDAY AUGUST 13

### TUESDAY AUGUST 14

### WEDNESDAY AUGUST 15

### THURSDAY AUGUST 16

### FRIDAY AUGUST 17

### SATURDAY AUGUST 18

### SUNDAY AUGUST 19

Weekly Planner

MONDAY **AUGUST 20**

TUESDAY **AUGUST 21**

WEDNESDAY **AUGUST 22**

THURSDAY **AUGUST 23**

FRIDAY **AUGUST 24**

SATURDAY **AUGUST 25**

SUNDAY **AUGUST 26**

# AUG 27-SEP 2 2018

MONDAY **AUGUST 27**

TUESDAY **AUGUST 28**

WEDNESDAY **AUGUST 29**

THURSDAY **AUGUST 30**

FRIDAY **AUGUST 31**

SATURDAY **SEPTEMBER 1**

SUNDAY **SEPTEMBER 2**

Weekly Planner

# SEPTEMBER 3-9

## MONDAY **SEPTEMBER 3**

## TUESDAY **SEPTEMBER 4**

## WEDNESDAY **SEPTEMBER 5**

## THURSDAY **SEPTEMBER 6**

## FRIDAY **SEPTEMBER 7**

## SATURDAY **SEPTEMBER 8**

## SUNDAY **SEPTEMBER 9**

# SEPTEMBER 10-16 — 2018

### MONDAY SEPTEMBER 10

### TUESDAY SEPTEMBER 11

### WEDNESDAY SEPTEMBER 12

### THURSDAY SEPTEMBER 13

### FRIDAY SEPTEMBER 14

### SATURDAY SEPTEMBER 15

### SUNDAY SEPTEMBER 16

# SEPTEMBER 17-23                    2018

**MONDAY  SEPTEMBER 17**

**TUESDAY  SEPTEMBER 18**

**WEDNESDAY  SEPTEMBER 19**

**THURSDAY  SEPTEMBER 20**

**FRIDAY  SEPTEMBER 21**

**SATURDAY  SEPTEMBER 22**

**SUNDAY  SEPTEMBER 23**

MONDAY **SEPTEMBER 24**

TUESDAY **SEPTEMBER 25**

WEDNESDAY **SEPTEMBER 26**

THURSDAY **SEPTEMBER 27**

FRIDAY **SEPTEMBER 28**

SATURDAY **SEPTEMBER 29**

SUNDAY **SEPTEMBER 30**

Weekly Planner

# OCTOBER 1-7 2018

MONDAY **OCTOBER 1**

TUESDAY **OCTOBER 2**

WEDNESDAY **OCTOBER 3**

THURSDAY **OCTOBER 4**

FRIDAY **OCTOBER 5**

SATURDAY **OCTOBER 6**

SUNDAY **OCTOBER 7**

MONDAY **OCTOBER 8**

TUESDAY **OCTOBER 9**

WEDNESDAY **OCTOBER 10**

THURSDAY **OCTOBER 11**

FRIDAY **OCTOBER 12**

SATURDAY **OCTOBER 13**

SUNDAY **OCTOBER 14**

Weekly Planner

# OCTOBER 15-21　　　2018

MONDAY **OCTOBER 15**

TUESDAY **OCTOBER 16**

WEDNESDAY **OCTOBER 17**

THURSDAY **OCTOBER 18**

FRIDAY **OCTOBER 19**

SATURDAY **OCTOBER 20**

SUNDAY **OCTOBER 21**

MONDAY **OCTOBER 22**

TUESDAY **OCTOBER 23**

WEDNESDAY **OCTOBER 24**

THURSDAY **OCTOBER 25**

FRIDAY **OCTOBER 26**

SATURDAY **OCTOBER 27**

SUNDAY **OCTOBER 28**

Weekly Planner

MONDAY **OCTOBER 29**

TUESDAY **OCTOBER 30**

WEDNESDAY **OCTOBER 31**

THURSDAY **NOVEMBER 1**

FRIDAY **NOVEMBER 2**

SATURDAY **NOVEMBER 3**

SUNDAY **NOVEMBER 4**

MONDAY **NOVEMBER 5**

TUESDAY **NOVEMBER 6**

WEDNESDAY **NOVEMBER 7**

THURSDAY **NOVEMBER 8**

FRIDAY **NOVEMBER 9**

SATURDAY **NOVEMBER 10**

SUNDAY **NOVEMBER 11**

Weekly Planner

# NOVEMBER 12-18　　2018

MONDAY **NOVEMBER 12**

TUESDAY **NOVEMBER 13**

WEDNESDAY **NOVEMBER 14**

THURSDAY **NOVEMBER 15**

FRIDAY **NOVEMBER 16**

SATURDAY **NOVEMBER 17**

SUNDAY **NOVEMBER 18**

# NOVEMBER 19-25 2018

MONDAY **NOVEMBER 19**

TUESDAY **NOVEMBER 20**

WEDNESDAY **NOVEMBER 21**

THURSDAY **NOVEMBER 22**

FRIDAY **NOVEMBER 23**

SATURDAY **NOVEMBER 24**

SUNDAY **NOVEMBER 25**

MONDAY **NOVEMBER 26**

TUESDAY **NOVEMBER 27**

WEDNESDAY **NOVEMBER 28**

THURSDAY **NOVEMBER 29**

FRIDAY **NOVEMBER 30**

SATURDAY **DECEMBER 1**

SUNDAY **DECEMBER 2**

MONDAY **DECEMBER 3**

TUESDAY **DECEMBER 4**

WEDNESDAY **DECEMBER 5**

THURSDAY **DECEMBER 6**

FRIDAY **DECEMBER 7**

SATURDAY **DECEMBER 8**

SUNDAY **DECEMBER 9**

Weekly Planner

MONDAY **DECEMBER 10**

TUESDAY **DECEMBER 11**

WEDNESDAY **DECEMBER 12**

THURSDAY **DECEMBER 13**

FRIDAY **DECEMBER 14**

SATURDAY **DECEMBER 15**

SUNDAY **DECEMBER 16**

## MONDAY **DECEMBER 17**

## TUESDAY **DECEMBER 18**

## WEDNESDAY **DECEMBER 19**

## THURSDAY **DECEMBER 20**

## FRIDAY **DECEMBER 21**

## SATURDAY **DECEMBER 22**

## SUNDAY **DECEMBER 23**

Weekly Planner

# DECEMBER 24-30

MONDAY **DECEMBER 24**

TUESDAY **DECEMBER 25**

WEDNESDAY **DECEMBER 26**

THURSDAY **DECEMBER 27**

FRIDAY **DECEMBER 28**

SATURDAY **DECEMBER 29**

SUNDAY **DECEMBER 30**

MONDAY **DECEMBER 31**

_____
_____
_____
_____
_____

# INDEX

Page numbers followed by *f* indicate figures, *b* indicate boxes, and *t* indicate tables.